Pink Warrior
Poetry & Tips

By

Karen E. Reid

First published in the USA by: Karen Reid

Paperback edition. 2015

© Copyright Karen Reid 2015
All rights reserved. No part of this book may be reproduced, stored in a retrieval system or transmitted in any form or by any means without the prior written permission of the publishers, except by a reviewer who may quote brief passages in a review to be printed in a newspaper, magazine or journal.

Available From:
Amazon.com
CreateSpace.com (https://www.createspace.com/5827972)
And other retail outlets

Cover Designed By: Stephanie Biddle at Corporate Imagination (Stephanie@corporateimagination.com)

The author can be contacted at: authorkreid@yahoo.com. She has also written *One Skater's Journey* and *Quest for Gold*.

Dedication

*To my husband,
the love of my life and my rock,
whose love and support
gave me the
mental and emotional fortitude
to survive this journey.*

*To my sister-in-law, dear friend,
cousin, and warriors before me…
For inspiring me to write
in honor of their personal fight.*

*And to my children,
who I love unconditionally.*

Table of Contents

Chapters

PREFACE……………………………..…................ 7
INTRODUCTION……………………………............ 8
AUTHOR'S STORY…………………….................. 11
    A Woman's Intuition 13
    Peer Poke & Prod 16
    My Journal 21
    Initial Assessment.. 24
    More Tests.. 30
    My D-Day (Diagnosis) 35
    And More Tests.. 38
    Battle Plan 42
    A Temporary Retreat... 45
    Surgery... 48
    Recovery.. 53
    Expect the Unexpected.. 58
    Symbolism.. 62
    Weighing the Options... 67
    Power of Prayer... 72
    One Two Punch.. 75
    In a Fog.. 76
    Healing... 78
    Finish Line 81
    Reflection... 85
    Live Love Laugh.. 93
    On the Bright Side... 101
    In Honor Of.. 104
    Concluding Thoughts 109
    All-Star Team 111

HELPFUL TIPS…....……………..…………….............. 120
AVAILABLE RESOURCES…....…………….....….......... 142
JOURNAL …..………………………………………........... 145

Table of Contents

Poems

Breast Cancer	10
The Journey	12
Tick Tock	22
Serenity	28
Bird Song	34
Cups of Love	44
Ladder of Life	49
The Beach	52
Shades of Pink	57
Pretty in Pink	61
Rainbows	72
Enlighten Me	74
Leather & Lace	76
Brain Freeze	78
Stitches	79
Pink Clouds	80
Reflection	87
Star Struck	100
Seasons	102
Think Pink	104
Mom	105
Grandmother	106
My Father…My Hero	107
Warrior	108
Soar High	110
Caregiver	113
A Mother's Touch	114
Dear Friend, My Sister	115
Pink Shawl	116
My Children	117
My Love	118

Preface

Pink Warrior Poetry & Tips is a personal story written by a cancer survivor who was inspired to write a collection of poems to capture her feelings as a patient who experienced the diagnosis and treatment of breast cancer. Through poetry she found an outlet to express herself and her story. In addition, the book includes tips from patients who have endured treatment and caregivers who wish to share their insight that may be helpful to someone newly diagnosed.

There is no clear roadmap to take one on this journey. Each individual will experience a process that may feel more like a maze with many twists and turns. It won't be easy; however, through the darkness will come light. From the time you are diagnosed, think of yourself as a survivor, and may this book give you the encouragement to fight like the warrior you will become.

As you turn the pages of this book, hopefully you will not feel alone, but rather, uplifted by someone who has battled this disease before you. Whether you use the book for inspiration or as a resource, may it bring a smile to your face and warm your heart to know that it was compiled with much love.

Introduction

Upon being diagnosed with breast cancer in November 2014, I started a journal. I never envisioned making my story into a book. My notes from doctor visits were meant to help keep me sane; while writing poetry became an outlet to voice my feelings in order to release the pain and give me a sense of peace.

As I embarked on the most difficult journey of my life, I was paralyzed with anxiety, not just by the diagnosis, but by the fact that there was no roadmap to explain how to maneuver one's way through the process. I didn't know what I didn't know, so figuring out who to call or what questions to ask was at times mind-numbing. Overnight, our lives were consumed with researching breast cancer. With insurance issues to deal with, doctors to research, delays in getting appointments as well as results, my life felt like a roller coaster ride out of control. The radiologist who told us to prepare for it, couldn't have been more accurate. Likewise, my sister-in-law and friend, who were also battling the disease at the same time, had their own set of challenges and experienced a similar level of anxiety.

A cancer diagnosis is overwhelming enough on its own. The process and timeframe to get the answers one seeks about their treatment should not be equally as scary. If my story and the tips that follow offer some guidance and help bring relief to even one patient, then it was worth documenting it.

Every year some 200,000+ women are diagnosed with breast cancer and approximately 40,000 die from it. The statistics are staggering, and the loss of life a tragedy. Please encourage your mothers, sisters, and friends to proactively get their annual mammograms. Approximately 80-85% of women diagnosed have no family history of the disease. It's true what they say…early detection saves lives. I sincerely hope and pray that a cure will be found for breast cancer during my lifetime.

BREAST CANCER

Beat the drums and make them listen
Rest not for the weary, as too many have risen
Embrace the light, and not the dark
Assume the fight, ignite a spark
Success will come if you believe
Together, we will achieve

Conquer this disease
Advocate for yourself and others…please
Nutrition is key to your well-being
Cope as the warrior that we are seeing
Encircle your loved ones and rally your supporters
Right from the start, you'll be one of many survivors

Author's Story

The Journey

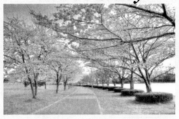

*Sometimes when we are faced
with problems it can be overwhelming,
especially when there doesn't seem
to be a solution in sight.*

*You may ask yourself, "Why me?"
It's a scary time and may seem
so unjust to be burdened
with such obstacles.*

*In life, the journey we take
may never be clear from peaks and
valleys, but eventually the path
will become smooth again.*

*If you believe in yourself
and focus on your dreams,
before long the future will
be full of promise.*

A Woman's Intuition

One morning in the gym a fellow member approached me and asked if I wanted to work out with her. Always open to changing up my workout routine, I happily accepted. For the next hour we lifted free weights working our upper body muscles (i.e. chest, biceps, triceps). It was challenging, but felt good. Not surprisingly, I was really sore the next day, but not anything I hadn't experienced before when modifying my routine; however, the pain continued for at least two to three weeks, especially in my chest to the point where my boobs really ached. These persistent aches got me thinking that there could be more to it than just normal muscle pain. When I reflect back on it now, I do believe that my body was giving me a wakeup call of sorts in order to explore the issue further. And, I did just that.

On Friday, November 7, 2014, I discovered a lump in my left breast. Honestly, I had never been one to do regular self-exams, but my sister-in-law (my husband's sister) had just finished chemotherapy for breast cancer. With my annual gynecology appointment scheduled three days away, even though breast cancer did not run in my immediate family, I felt compelled to check. I was astonished to find a hard knot on the side of my breast that did not move. It felt like finding a pebble in the sand about the size of a nickel. Although I kept telling myself it could be a cyst or a benign tumor, my intuition told me there was something wrong. This was the start of my own journey with breast cancer.

For three days, I anxiously awaited my doctor's appointment. I did some research on the web and learned that breast pain was a possible symptom of breast cancer. I kept feeling the lump to see if it would move, hoping it was just a cyst, but it definitely was stationary. Not to worry my family, I didn't say anything. I tried to keep myself as busy as possible. Perhaps if I ignored it, it would miraculously go away. When Monday, November 10th finally arrived, the wait to see the doctor seemed liked hours. Extremely nervous, I tried to fill the time by reading the latest gossip magazines in the waiting room, but all I could do was stare at the same story and read the same sentence over and over again. I looked around the room and wondered who else might be feeling the same level of panic inside. There were several pregnant women who reminded me of happier of times, and there were younger women who appeared quite calm. I was consumed with fear and just wanted to stand up and scream, but instead I held it together. When I finally was called into the exam room, I explained to the doctor what I had felt. As soon as she examined me, she felt it too. I could see the concerned look on her face. She immediately wrote a script for a 3-D mammogram and ultrasound. Her office manager was able to get me an appointment the very next day, but it wasn't until 6 o'clock at night. It was going to be a very long torturous 24 hours, but first I had to tell my husband what was happening.

Given the circumstances, I gave myself the best pep talk I knew how all the way home in the car...*think positive, think positive thoughts only, everything will be okay.* As strong as I wanted to be, as soon as I saw him I broke down, so much for trying to keep a stiff upper-lip! He was so confused at first because I caught him completely off guard. I felt guilty for not telling him about the lump that I had found, but I wanted to protect him so he wouldn't worry. He held me close and did the best he could to try and reassure me that everything would be fine, that the doctor was probably just being extra cautious and that more than likely it would be nothing. My inner voice spoke to me, softly at first...*What were the chances, right?* And then it was louder...***It didn't run in my family.***

Peer Poke & Prod

On November 11, 2014 I went to a local radiology center for my tests. Just like in years past, I sat in the waiting area tied up in my pink surgical gown surrounded by other women. No one spoke, just sat there quietly waiting, wondering (*what if*), and courteously respecting each other's privacy. The sound of the clock ticking and TV blaring were simply background noise to fill the void. I stared at the TV hoping to engage in one of my favorite shows (HGTV), but I was unable to focus. To my left, on a table, was a pamphlet about breast cancer. I instinctively picked it up. The first detail that caught my attention was a statistic that estimated about 1 in 8 women on average develops the disease. *A frightening statistic*…I thought to myself. I quickly folded and returned the pamphlet to its proper place. I took a deep breath in, and a huge exhale out. Suddenly, I heard my name being called. Rather than run, I dutifully stood, smiled and followed the technician down the hall.

First, I had a 3-D mammogram which took about the same amount of time as a regular mammogram. Next, I was escorted to a different room for the ultrasound. I had mixed emotions about having an ultrasound. Out of the four I had experienced in years past, two had provided the most beautiful images of our unborn children; while two images indicated there were complications. Blessed to eventually deliver two healthy children, we also mourned the two we lost. Once again, this machine would determine my fate...

Since the area of concern was with my left breast, the technician started there. At first, she seemed to scan the area just watching the monitor, but after a few minutes had passed she began to click away taking picture after picture and measurements. The silence was agonizing. I knew there was no point in verbalizing my thoughts and asking what she saw as it would be the radiologist who would have to deliver the outcome of the tests. Finally, she finished and excused herself to take the results to the doctor. About 10 minutes later, the technician returned to the room and explained that the doctor wanted her to take some pictures of the right breast for comparisons. She apologized and while she tried her best to make this seem like standard protocol, I had a sinking feeling that my situation had gone from bad to worse. Again, she began clicking away. I stared at the clock on the wall at the foot of the examining table. As much as I tried to think positive thoughts, I knew I had to prepare myself for the worst case scenario. *But what had she found?* I lied still as a statue trying to disconnect myself from the situation. If I didn't feel, then the news wouldn't hurt so badly. I didn't ask, *"Why me?"* as that question has no answer and only brings your mental and emotional psyche down. I was focused more on how this might affect my family. Soon enough, some of my questions would be answered.

After what seemed like an eternity, the testing was complete. *Did I pass? Tests were always about pass or fail, right?* I had always been good at taking tests, but this one was out my control. As I sat waiting for the doctor, I looked at the ultrasound screen trying to make sense of what it might tell me, but I quickly realized I had no idea. Once the doctor reviewed both the 3-D mammogram and ultrasound results, she knocked on the door.

The room was dimly lit, brightened only by the glow from the monitor on the ultrasound equipment. Per my insistence, my husband had stayed home with our son so my late doctor's appointment wouldn't raise any suspicions; therefore, at my request, I called my husband to conference him in to the discussion. As I sat just a few feet away from the doctor, the look on her face confirmed that I needed to brace myself for bad news. While it was reassuring to hear my husband's voice, I felt like a lone soldier being shot when she delivered the results. The tests showed that there were actually 2 tumors in my left breast and 1 in my right. As she continued to talk, my head was spinning and trying to process this information. *What did she say? Did I hear her say 3? How could there be 3? Why did these go undetected?* I had always gotten my mammograms. Shaken to the core, I gripped the table next to me afraid to let go. I could hear my husband asking questions, and the doctor explaining the next steps to further identify the types of tumors and whether or not they were malignant or benign. It was too soon to tell exactly what we were dealing with, but she felt that they were caught early because nothing had been detected on previous mammograms. The one tumor I had initially found appeared to be of most concern to her and she told us to prepare ourselves for a potential rollercoaster ride. Our next step was to schedule an appointment to biopsy each of the tumors.

It took all my strength to try and maintain my composure. I remember tearing up and thinking that I needed to get out of there. I felt like I was suffocating and couldn't speak, yet I managed to mumble something inaudible like, "*I knew this was not going to be good, I had a feeling, I just knew it. Thank you for your time doctor.*" I quickly dressed and escaped into the cool night air. It was strangely silent and completely dark, not a star in the sky. As I slammed my fists on the steering wheel in my car, I felt overwhelmed by a plethora of emotions. I prayed that God would give me the strength to bravely deal with whatever happened next.

As I sat frozen, I was startled by the ring of my phone. I knew before I looked that it would be my husband. When I answered, he said, "It will be okay. I love you. Are you alright to drive?" Choked up, I managed to say, "*Yes*". "Please come home," he said. All I could verbalize was "*okay*".

I felt like a dark cloud was hovering and followed me all the way home. When I walked in the door there were no words exchanged between us. My husband hugged me tight and we both exploded with emotion. It was as if a hurricane had swooped in to our lives with gale force winds without warning. It was disorienting, as if the world had suddenly becomes a different place. Would we be able to weather this storm? His love gave me reassurance that night that somehow everything would be alright.

My Journal

The next day I decided to start a journal to document my appointments and the anguish I was feeling inside. I felt it was the only way to help keep me sane through what was about to become the most difficult journey of my life. As I sat down at my desk, I felt compelled to write a poem. Other than probably grade school, I had never seriously written poetry before in my life. I figured I would write one, share it with my husband, and be done. Although I didn't know it then, poetry would become an outlet for me over the coming months as a means for me to voice my feelings about certain events during my journey. Without hesitation, the words just flowed. Whether or not it was any good, didn't matter to me, I didn't think anyone but my husband would see it. I carried that journal from one appointment to the next. At times, I was inspired to write while sitting in a waiting room. It became therapeutic to write. The poem ***Tick Tock*** would be the first of many to follow.

Tick Tock

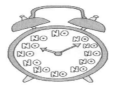

*Tick tock, tick tock
I patiently watched the movement of the clock*

*It was exactly six o'clock
I sat fixated in a trance…as still as a rock*

*Perhaps if I didn't move, think or feel
This situation would somehow become unreal*

*Many a times I had sat in this very waiting room
But never did I feel my fate loom*

*As the TV projected my favorite show
All I could hear from my inner voice was…**"get up and go"***

*Instead I sat frozen, tied up like a bow
Mentally stressed and emotionally low*

*The day before I found a lump in my chest
These tests would put any questions to rest*

*So there I sat in my pink surgical robe
My ears ringing from lobe to lobe…**"get up and go"***

*Perhaps it would be a cyst or a benign tumor
But all I could focus on was that scary word **"cancer"***

*Looking for answers, I reached for a pamphlet
It mentioned a woman's circle of eight*

*One in eight women are diagnosed with breast cancer each year
If this was my fate, then I prayed my intimate circle would be spared*

*The technician arrived and called out my name
I dutifully stood and told myself, **"I'm game"***

*Mammogram and ultrasound, what did I have to fear?
This didn't run in my family, as I fought to hold back a tear*

*As the technicians diligently snapped their pictures
All I could think about…were my sisters*

"Sisters"... family, friends and strangers
How many had come before me mentally consumed by the same dangers?

Now as I laid there awaiting my result
The doctor would ultimately provide the final consult

Time was moving forward and getting so late
Usually calm, but I was getting a bit irate

My head began to spin...I was panicked, angry and filled with deep sadness
The waiting was killing me, this simply was madness

I could hear my own breath as I laid quietly in the dim of the light
Finally, the doctor appeared at the door all dressed in white

Her movements were delicate, but her face cold as stone
I knew then what was coming, and I felt so alone

As she delivered the news...not one, nor two, but three tumors found
If I hadn't gripped the table, I would have crumbled to the ground

So there it was, out in the air
It will be a rollercoaster ride, you need to prepare

My instinct was right before I heard even a word
But her delivery cut to my gut like a sword

So many questions (What?, How?, Why?) filled my head
But nothing seemed clear, I was numb with disbelief and my brain just went dead

Stage one, two, three, or four
It was just too soon to score

There was mention of next steps and the journey ahead
But all I could focus on was my family instead

I quickly dressed and exited the door
When I got in my car I yelled to the Lord

I slammed my fist on the wheel and begged him for the courage to fight
But I would need his guidance to do what was right

In a daze, I found my way home to the love of my life
For soon I would add "warrior" to my title of mother and wife

As I looked into his worried, yet loving eyes
He assured me he'd move heaven and earth so that I would not die

You see, ours is a love story that spans thirty-two years
He's my partner, my lover, my best friend... who truly cares

That night I lay my head on my pillow and offered up grace
I put my faith in God's hands and my husband's warm embrace

Initial Assessment

Within a few days of my 3-D mammogram and ultrasound, I would learn that I had heterogeneously dense breasts. A term I had never heard mentioned in the ten years I had been going for mammograms. Unbeknownst to me, the state of New Jersey had passed a law earlier in the year requiring that all mammography reports sent to patients and their physicians provide an assessment of your breast density. There are 4 categories: A. Predominantly fatty; B. Scattered fibrograndular; C. Heterogeneously dense; and D. Extremely dense. According to my gynecologist, heterogeneously dense breasts were considered quite common and did not increase my chances of breast cancer. It may not have increased my chances, but I would always wonder if that's why the tumors went undetected on previous tests. I read that both cancer and dense breast tissue look white or light gray on a mammogram; therefore, dense tissue may hide a tumor from view.

Initially, I was given a date for the biopsies three weeks out from my meeting with the radiologist. The scheduler told me that it was the earliest date available. My husband and I were shocked. We called my gynecologist's office to see if they could assist with expediting the process. They were able to move the date, but I would still have to wait two weeks. Never did my husband or I ever feel so helpless. We were both problem solvers. Our mode of operation was always…if you had an issue, you fixed it. However, this was out of our control and we didn't even know where to begin. With all the media attention and fundraisers for breast cancer awareness, how could it be that when you found yourself diagnosed there was no one knocking at your door to guide you through this process? I never felt so helpless in my life. I was at a complete loss as to which way to turn. My husband reached out to his sister for guidance, but what we learned very early on was that the protocol and response time for treatment seemed to vary depending upon your State, hospital, doctors, prognosis, etc. Our level of anxiety was off the charts. Basically, we were on our own treading water and waiting for someone to throw us a life vest.

While we waited for the biopsy date to arrive, per the recommendation of my gynecologist, we scheduled a visit with a local breast surgeon. Once again, we hit another obstacle with scheduling a date. When I called the doctor's office I was given an appointment two months out. **Two months?!** I thought to myself…*this is insane, I might have* **CANCER!** I felt like my life was a pendulum swinging between hope and despair. Disheartened, I accepted the date, but immediately got back on the phone with my gynecologist's office to see, what if anything, could be done to better this date. Fortunately, the office manager was able to get me an appointment with another surgeon three days after my ultrasound.

The night before my appointment with the breast surgeon, I was extremely restless. I did my best to put on a brave face during the day, but anxiety crept in when night fell and it was time to sleep. It was November 13th (which happens to be my deceased father's birthday), the sixth night in a row that I just couldn't sleep. I tossed and turned watching the clock. Around 2AM, I began to pray…for guidance, for a healing, for courage, and for sleep!

As I finally fell off to sleep from exhaustion, I had a dream. In the dream, strange as it may sound, I found myself swimming with whale sharks. At first, it was scary, as I felt myself sinking deeper into the depths of the ocean and I couldn't breathe. The light illuminating the surface was drifting further away as I drifted deeper, but there was a shift in my breathing. I went from fighting to survive to being overcome with peace. The next thing I knew, I was swimming along side of two whale sharks. Their enormous size and power was intimidating, but I felt they were protecting me as a mother and father would do for their child. We swam through the darkness and it was so serene. Ninety-five percent of the time I never remember my dreams, but this one was so vivid, I couldn't forget it.

Two years prior we had gone on a family vacation to Mexico and swam with whale sharks in the ocean. They are the most beautiful enormous peaceful creatures. This was the one and only time the whale sharks appeared in a dream for me. When I awoke the next morning, it was the first time in seven days that I had a sense of calmness, that somehow I would be okay. That day I wrote *Serenity*.

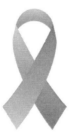

Serenity

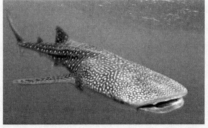

My body physically tossed and turned in a thrashing feat
Mentally unaware of my calming heart beat

Darkness enveloped me, it was scary at first
Blindly finding my way, it was air that I thirst

As I focused my vision
I was shocked by my position

Sandwiched between a mother and father
Two whale sharks coddling me like a toddler

Although our direction seemed virtually unknown
I trusted their compass to help find my way home

We swam through the ocean with power and ease
Awed by their strength, putting me at peace

The passing waves made the sound of a womb
A tranquil feeling liked being wrapped in a cocoon

This overwhelming feeling of comfort, safety and love
Made it difficult to want to rise above

But when I awoke, the feelings of hopelessness and despair
Began to slip away, I could manage these fears

I would read that poem over several times that day, both before my doctor's appointment, and especially after it, to calm my nerves. When we arrived at the surgeon's office we were told that they didn't accept our insurance. Apparently, the electronic referral did not transmit successfully from my gynecologist to the surgeon's office. As if possibly having cancer wasn't stressful enough, now we had to deal with insurance coverage issues. We called the insurance company from the doctor's office, but there was no negotiating any coverage for a doctor who was considered out-of-network. This stand-off with the insurance company would set off a flurry of activity for the next three weeks trying to research alternative insurance options for us. Desperate, we opted to see the doctor and pay cash so we could speak with someone to assess my situation.

I was shocked to learn that approximately 80-85% of women who develop breast cancer have no family history of it, just like me. Although the biopsy would be key to understanding exactly what we were dealing with, the doctor took a look at my mammography films from the last 3 years. Her initial assessment was that the tumor in my right didn't appear to be worrisome. As for the two in my left, they were in different quadrants; therefore, if one was malignant, she would recommend a lumpectomy with partial reconstruction. If both tumors were malignant, the recommendation would be a mastectomy, but either way, she assured us that these appeared to be small tumors that were caught early and that regardless of the outcome, I would be okay. My husband sat across from me, so still and pale, that when the doctor turned from examining me and saw his face, she ever so gently touched his shoulder and again said, "She's going to be okay, I promise." That was the first time in seven days that anyone made us feel like it really was going to be okay and that it didn't appear to be a life or death situation. She took the time to explain what the next steps would be after the biopsy and even gave me a hug before leaving the office. Sadly, I left her office knowing that a really special doctor had just slipped through our hands because of our insurance policy.

More Tests

Two weeks seemed like two years, but the day finally arrived for my biopsy. We returned to the same radiology center and the same doctor. Although my husband couldn't be in the room during the procedure, he paced in the waiting room till I was finished.

The radiologist performed three ultrasound-guided biopsies. The vacuum-assisted device was a bit noisy, a little unsettling, and the needle attached to it looked like something out of the movie Ghostbusters used to extinguish the ghosts. I thought to myself, *if the needle is that big why not extract the entire tumor and save me the aggravation and months of torture?* The answer to this question would soon become clear. Using the ultrasound as her guide to find the exact locations of each tumor, she numbed the areas and utilized the needle to extract tissue samples from the core of each one. Once the areas were numb, I really didn't feel much. Only when she inserted a small metal clip into two of the three tumors, I felt a slight pinch. It was explained that this was done to mark the sites so they could be spotted easily on future mammograms. After the procedure was complete, they did another mammogram so they would have the latest films on file.

My husband was invited back to the room and a nurse provided us some guidelines on how to treat the areas over the coming days (i.e. pain medication, icing the areas, signs of infection). Although Thanksgiving was the following week, they assured us that the test would be marked STAT to try and expedite the results before the long holiday weekend.

I went back to work that afternoon with ice packs in my bra. As a figure skating coach it was uncomfortable moving around the ice, but I needed the diversion. Working with my students always put me in a good mood. Besides, what kind of coach would I be if I gave up and quit in the eyes of adversity? Just like I expected them to work hard and persevere, now it was my turn to fight. Cancer was not going to stop me from a profession that I loved.

Impatiently, we awaited the results. Within 24 hours my chest looked like I had gone ten rounds in a boxing ring. I have a tendency to bruise easily, so I was very swollen and extremely black and blue. This was to be expected, but shocking nevertheless.

Over the weekend, I took our dog outside for a walk. I felt like the fresh air would help me to breath and clear my head. While on our walk, I was distracted by a red cardinal. Although I know cardinals are a common bird, I hadn't seen one by our house in years. For some reason, he seemed determined to get my attention. At one point, he flew right by my head and made me jump because he was so close. His wing actually brushed my ear. After darting from tree to tree, he finally landed on a bare limb right in front of me. He started chirping up a storm. He was so loud, I couldn't believe my dog didn't start barking at him, but he seemed more occupied with sniffing the ground. I don't know why, but at that moment, I felt there was something special about this bird. If only for a few minutes, I was mesmerized by him. Almost as quick as he had arrived distracting me from my thoughts, he fluttered past me and took off out of sight.

 Although I'm not typically one to be superstitious or analyze situations for hidden meanings, I mention this bird because the cardinal was one of two species that would play a significant role in my story. ***Bird Song*** was penned as a result of this cardinal visit.

Bird Song

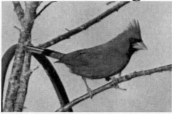

Days after receiving the news,
I sought solace with nature heeding our dog's cues

The silence was welcoming
But the noise in my head was deafening

I stood in the middle of the road
Trying to make sense of the code

Red, yellow, or green
So many twists and turns in between

If I turned left or right
Would there be a miracle in sight?

"Cheer, cheer", I heard it so clear
He missed me by inches as he brushed by my ear

He flitted and fluttered from branch to branch
Making sure I watched his elegant dance

I looked up and quickly down
There he perched with his fiery crown

Determined to keep my attention
His powerful presence certainly made an impression

His color was bold against the bare tree
Crimson red, a symbol of strength; was it a key for me?

Perhaps he was sent as a reminder of steadfast faith
That even through dark times, he would somehow keep me safe

As I stood dumb-founded, stricken with grief and depression
This bird brought me hope and a feeling of self-preservation

In all his glory, he suddenly took flight
Upward he soared escaping my sight

Although his visit ever so brief
He awoke a spirit that ignited some relief

And so I've been told…when cardinals appear
Do not fear, it's a sign that angels are near

My D-Day (Diagnosis)

While waiting for the biopsy results, I began to research other doctors covered by our plan (just in case we couldn't switch companies), as well as other insurance carriers. Once again, I referred back to my gynecologist's office for additional references for breast surgeons. They recommended a group associated with a large well-known cancer research and teaching hospital about thirty minutes away. It didn't help matters that we got lost on the way to our first appointment. Nervous enough to begin with, by the time we arrived, I was shaking like a leaf, my mouth was dry, and my heart was practically beating out of my chest. I thought for sure if everyone was silent around me that they would hear it.

My pathology report was back on my biopsies and I found myself sitting with a new breast surgeon. Overwhelmed by the list of acronyms, our initial meeting felt more like a military summit where cancer was the enemy and I was the defender, and our battle plan would be based on how far the enemy had infiltrated my territory. There were more codes to decipher than an artillery strategy from the Pentagon.

The one tumor in my right breast was benign…*a sigh of relief.* However, the two tumors located in my left breast were of two different types of cancers: invasive ductal carcinoma (IDC) and ductal carcinoma in situ (DCIS). IDC starts by developing in the milk ducts of your breast, but breaks out of the duct tubes, and invades surrounding tissues. Unlike DCIS which is a non-invasive cancer, IDC is not a well-contained cancer. IDC has the potential to invade your lymph and blood systems, spreading cancer cells to other parts of your body. The keys to my treatment would be determined by the stage of the cancer, grade of the tumors, hormone receptor results, HER2 oncogene results, and whether or not it had spread to my lymph nodes. It was too early to stage without further tests; however, she felt that it was caught early because it hadn't appeared on previous mammograms. Each tumor was a grade 2 (out of 3). Since my lymph node area felt swollen, the doctor ordered an MRI to get a more detailed look at the areas in question with a possible node biopsy.

In addition, my estrogen and progesterone levels were positive (ER+ and PR+) which meant that receptors for both of these types of hormones were detected in a significant number of the cancer cells in the breast tissue. And my HER2 oncogene test was negative (HER2-) which meant that, these types of cancer would be more cooperative when it came to various treatments (i.e. hormone therapy, chemotherapy). It was a lot of information to absorb. Thank goodness my husband took meticulous notes because we would find ourselves referring back to these over the coming weeks. Per her initial assessment, because the tumors were in different quadrants, the recommendation was for me to have a mastectomy. Questions regarding chemotherapy and radiation would have to wait until more tests were run and we met with an oncologist. It was too soon to tell definitively what may/may not be needed.

Our new doctor had many years of experience, she was the head of the department at the hospital, and she was extremely patient with answering all of our questions. We felt very confident with her credentials, her disposition and her extremely helpful staff. Over the following weeks, her nurse navigator would become like a big sister to me, holding my hand through the process and keeping me sane when it came to trying to understand all the medical terminology and procedures being discussed. Moreover, her nurse practitioner always made my appointments as pleasant as possible with her kind temperament.

That night, for the first time in years, totally out of the blue, my son crawled into bed to snuggle with me. At first I thought he was trying to extend his bedtime on a school night, but he assured me he didn't come to watch TV, just to sleep. Rather than argue, I put my arm around him and let him curl up next to me. He may not have known it then, but it felt good to have him close to me. Mentally and emotionally drained, I needed more than anything the love and support of my family. I held on extra tight that night.

And More Tests

Prior to having the MRI, we felt, and with the affirmation from our doctor, that we needed to share what was happening with our children. Our daughter was eighteen and our son was twelve. Since it was Thanksgiving, our daughter was home from college so the timing seemed right. Do to the flurry of doctors' calls and follow up appointments, my son knew something was up. Rather than delay the inevitable, now that we had a sense of next steps, we felt it was time to share the news. Next to my husband, this was the second most difficult conversation I would have about my diagnosis. The fact that my sister-in-law had breast cancer helped us to ease in to the discussion. Both of our children had spent enough time around their aunt during her treatment to know that she had handled it well and remained in good spirits throughout her ordeal. Still, when we sat down, I had my husband lead the discussion because my emotions were just too raw. I wanted to be strong so they wouldn't worry. As I looked at their faces all I could think about were their dreams and big moments ahead...*graduations, weddings, grandchildren, etc.* I couldn't imagine a future without being there for them. It was not an easy discussion, but they were old enough to fully grasp the situation and were prepared to deal with our next steps. I know it was scary for them too, but I was consoled by their strength and would fight for all three of them.

The MRI, which was done on November 28th, indicated that the cancer appeared to be contained in the breast area; however, they still recommended a lymph node biopsy. Five days later I had the biopsy done, and two days after that, on December 5th, my radiologist and surgeon called to share the good news. The nodes tested were clear. As the lymph nodes are the gateway to the rest of your body, this was a call for a short-lived celebration because early indicators were that the cancer had not spread beyond my breasts. Given these results, along with the tumor grades, hormone receptors and oncogene indicators, it did not appear that chemotherapy would be necessary **prior** to surgery. The overall assessment was that I had an early form of multifocal (more than 1) invasive carcinoma (malignant tumors), possibly stage 1 or 2.

A few days later, we had a consultation with the chief of oncology and a genetic counselor at the same hospital. Our feeling of elation was momentarily dashed when we learned that a negative core biopsy of the lymph nodes could still end up positive during surgery. Having to accept the limitations of some of these tests that I entrusted with my life was frustrating, confusing and made me angry. She went on to explain that during the operation, the surgeon would extract a sentinel node (aka. frozen section). Upon extraction, the entire lymph node (not just a tissue sample) would be sent to pathology for immediate review. If the result of testing was negative, then that would confirm that the cancer hadn't spread. If the result was positive, the surgeon would remove anxillary nodes, in an effort to further stop the spread of the disease. Until the operation was completed, it was too soon to determine whether or not I would need either chemotherapy or radiation post-surgery. The type of hormone therapy treatment would be decided after surgery as well.

The oncologist had us meet with a genetic counselor to discuss my family medical history, both immediate and extended. Even though no one in my immediate family had had breast cancer, I did have a cousin who had survived stage 3-4. Since I had a benign tumor in my right breast, I was very concerned about the cancer possibly recurring; therefore, the counselor suggested that I submit a blood sample to test for the BRCA 1 and BRCA 2 gene mutations (these are the two most common inherited breast cancer genes). The results of this test would let me know if I was a carrier of the gene(s) that may have initiated the breast cancer. This would not only be important to my daughter for future testing, but the doctors felt that it might help me to make my decision with whether to do a single or double mastectomy. If I decided to go with a single mastectomy, I would have 3-D mammograms and ultrasounds for the remainder of my life in order to catch any recurrence at an early stage. My doctors assured me that I would be watched closely; however, I would have to decide in the end what would be best for me. This decision loomed large as I needed to decide whether or not I could mentally handle the stress of always wondering and waiting to see if breast cancer would return. Eight days later I would receive a call indicating that the test came back negative for both genes. Although this was a huge relief to my husband and to some degree myself, I still couldn't sleep at night.

Battle Plan

While I continued to mull over my decision, we met with a plastic surgeon who specialized in breast reconstruction. We discussed my options, but in the end, he felt that I would be most satisfied with the outcome by doing back latissimus dorsi flap surgery with an implant. Basically, the breast reconstruction is done using the diagonal muscle and surrounding fat that's located on the side of your back, behind the armpit. A small incision is made along the bra strap line to hide any potential scar from surgery. The flap is then slipped from the back to the front. Because the muscle is fairly small and there's little body fat in that area an implant would be necessary to complete the reconstruction. Post-surgery, I would have a tissue expander(s) (one or two depending on a single or double mastectomy) which would be filled over time to achieve my desired size. Future surgery would be completed to swap the expander(s) out for an implant(s). Not having any medical training I had no choice but to lean on the experts for their opinion as to what made the most sense given my situation. I was beginning to feel like I was in a maze in the dark trying to find my way to the next open doorway. My breast surgeon and reconstructive doctors became my guides to get me to the finish line, so I could see the light again. They both were in agreement that this would be the best solution for me. We were confident that after intense research and discussions that we had assembled an outstanding team to help navigate us through the process.

A bit uncomfortable with too much attention, especially under serious circumstances, I often try to find ways to lighten the conversation, especially with doctors. Our first meeting with the reconstructive doctor was one such occasion…serious and informative, but when the doctor went to leave the room I stopped him and said, *"Wait, when do we discuss how big I'd like to be?"* He smiled courteously and said, "There's plenty of time to discuss that don't worry." *"Can you promise me cleavage?"* I replied. He laughed and said, "Yes, as big as you'd like." Perhaps it sounds shallow, but it was the silver lining during a really dark time. It wasn't meant to be crude or disrespectful, but rather, in a small way it offered me comfort.

By the time I left his office, I felt like my head would

implode with all the information I needed to digest from over the last couple of weeks. Oddly enough, it didn't stop me from reading more books, researching information on-line, and talking to breast cancer survivors. This served to raise even more questions which I leaned on my nurse navigator for answers. She was extremely knowledgeable and very patient with me, even when I called her back with the same question multiple times.

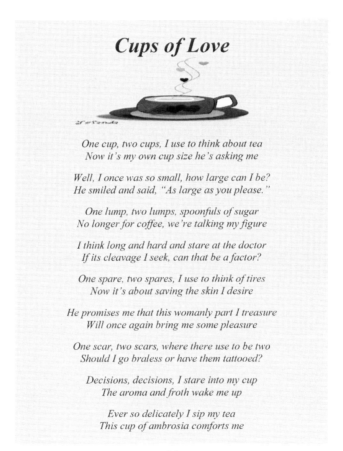

Cups of Love

One cup, two cups, I use to think about tea
Now it's my own cup size he's asking me

Well, I once was so small, how large can I be?
He smiled and said, "As large as you please."

One lump, two lumps, spoonfuls of sugar
No longer for coffee, we're talking my figure

I think long and hard and stare at the doctor
If its cleavage I seek, can that be a factor?

One spare, two spares, I use to think of tires
Now it's about saving the skin I desire

He promises me that this womanly part I treasure
Will once again bring me some pleasure

One scar, two scars, where there use to be two
Should I go braless or have them tattooed?

Decisions, decisions, I stare into my cup
The aroma and froth wake me up

Ever so delicately I sip my tea
This cup of ambrosia comforts me

A Temporary Retreat

By mid-December I was given a date of January 9th for my surgery. My heart sank as this was the same timeframe that my son was expected to be in Canada for a hockey tournament. With my health hanging in the balance, my focus shifted to my son. My stress level went up ten-fold. I certainly didn't want him to have to miss out on such an exciting experience, and it pained me to know that if he went that I would not be present to cheer him and his teammates on. My husband reasoned that perhaps this was a blessing in disguise…with our daughter away at school it might be better for our son to be out of town the same weekend as my surgery too. Without hesitation several families were willing to help and offered to take our son with them to Canada. So a plan was set in motion to have him travel with another hockey family while I underwent surgery. No sooner did we cancel our reservations and get everything set for our son when we were thrown another curve ball. My plastic surgeon was unavailable; so we found ourselves back in a holding pattern waiting on a date when all the stars would align…availability of the operating room, my breast surgeon and plastic surgeon.

On December 23, 2014, my doctor's office called with a new surgery date of January 19, 2015…ten weeks after I found a lump. While my husband was panicking that this might be taking too long, for fear that the cancer might spread; I was consumed with making a life-altering decision about my body and my future. I was extremely fortunate that my husband was very supportive and voiced that he would be fine with whatever choice I made. Our love was strong, like any relationship we had endured our own trials and tribulations over the years, but a cancer diagnosis can test a relationship in so many ways; he assured me that our relationship was solid and professed his love for me on a daily basis. It pained me to see how distraught with fear he was for my health, but at the same time it was also comforting to feel the depth of his love. Although it was my body infected with cancer, I knew that he would be supportive of whatever decision I made. I needed to do some serious soul searching to be very sure (as confident as I could be) with my final decision. During the day, I would go about keeping myself busy with work, only allowing the lingering question to creep in when I had a lull in activity. At night, I would toss and turn watching the clock and replay every conversation over the last two months trying to decide what to do. The doctors felt that this was caught early…they were relatively small in size, slow growing, low grade tumors and the lymph node had tested negative as well as the BRCA test. With no family history, their only explanation was that it was probably caused by the environment. *The environment, what did that mean?* Possibly anything and everything from diet (*Had I consumed too much red meat and processed food?*), to drinking (*I stuck mostly to wine as my choice of alcohol which most doctors will say is fine.*), to stress (*Did I harbor too much inside?*), to the start of menstruation (*I was twelve like most of my friends, not too young.*), to my age during pregnancies (*I was in my 30's, had I waited too long?*), to not breastfeeding (*Which I did not.*), to timing of menopause (*Which I hadn't yet experienced.*), etc. All of these thoughts were running through my head like a ticker tape. *Had I caused this?* The guilt was unbearable despite the fact that doctors, nurses, and everything I read said "*no*". There was no rhyme or reason as to why, it just happened. *Cancer just happened.*

We did our best to try and enjoy the Christmas holiday by going through the motions of our annual family traditions. At an attempt to escape everything "cancer", we took a family retreat to Florida to visit my mom. Some desperately needed family bonding time was just what the doctor ordered.

Once we returned home, the waiting period tested every ounce of my patience, but there was still more work to be done (i.e. EKG, blood work). I busied myself with work and getting things ready for our son's trip. He was over the moon excited to go; while I grew more depressed about not being able to go. Even though my surgery date had been moved out, it was too late to re-book accommodations and I still needed to get things in order for my new surgery date. As it turned out, he had a fabulous time. Their team won the tournament. In addition, his essay was selected as the winner for his division which earned him a free week at summer hockey camp. The text messages, pictures and phone calls kept coming from multiple families. As the good news emerged, I didn't know whether to scream, laugh or cry. I was so thrilled for him and his team. It saddened me not to be there with him to celebrate his accomplishments, but at the same time I was overjoyed for them. Their victory was a welcome divergence from everything else going on in our lives.

Surgery

You never know how strong you are until being strong is the only choice you have... By January 12th, I had to give my doctors a decision regarding my surgery. After extensive research, discussions with my husband and other cancer survivors, and prayer, I elected to proceed with a double mastectomy. The advances in reconstructive surgery, and not having to stress about future mammograms, helped me to make the single most difficult decision I had ever made in my life. For peace of mind, I felt it was the best choice for my personal situation… *I was ready to move forward.*

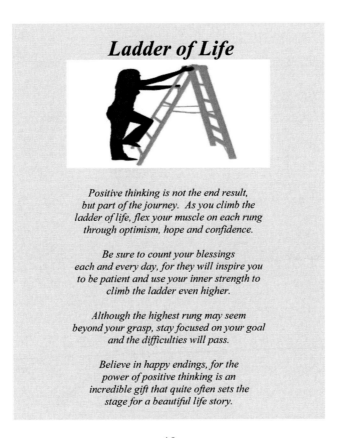

Ladder of Life

*Positive thinking is not the end result,
but part of the journey. As you climb the
ladder of life, flex your muscle on each rung
through optimism, hope and confidence.*

*Be sure to count your blessings
each and every day, for they will inspire you
to be patient and use your inner strength to
climb the ladder even higher.*

*Although the highest rung may seem
beyond your grasp, stay focused on your goal
and the difficulties will pass.*

*Believe in happy endings, for the
power of positive thinking is an
incredible gift that quite often sets the
stage for a beautiful life story.*

Approximately one week prior to surgery, I met with my breast surgeon's nurse practitioner to sign off on paperwork for the operation, as well as to discuss more details about the surgery. First, she mentioned that a dye would be injected into the areola to help the doctor locate the lymph node to be extracted and tested. Next, she used an avocado as an analogy. She explained that the surgery was similar to slicing an avocado in half and scooping out the innards. The seed inside the avocado would be like the tumor inside the breast tissue. Both the tissue (innards) and tumors (seed) would be sent to pathology for analysis. Since I was having skin-sparring mastectomies, the outer layer of the breasts would be left intact once the reconstructive doctor completed the back latissimus surgery and inserted tissue expanders. After all the research I had done, this was probably the best (and least technical) explanation anyone had given me which I really appreciated.

When the day for surgery finally arrived I was somewhat relieved, but apprehensive at the same time. Over two months had passed since my initial diagnosis. While I was confident in my choice of doctors and my decision to have a double mastectomy, my fear of the unknown post-surgery caused my blood pressure to sky-rocket to 210/99. Since November, it had been steadily rising from my normal range of 130/70. Fortunately, the anesthesiologist gave me medication to help control my blood pressure prior to surgery.

As the nurse started my IV, I noticed a picture of the beach that hung on the wall. It was beautiful and I remember wishing that I was there instead. My husband caught my gaze and said, "When this is all behind us and you're feeling up to it, we'll get away to the beach. I promise." True to his word, we would return to one of our favorite travel destinations eight months later.

Both my breast and plastic surgeons visited with me before surgery. They reassured us that everything would be fine. For a fleeting moment I was scared to death, but when my breast surgeon hugged my mother, her kind gesture touched my heart and a sense of calmness came over me. I kissed my mother and husband and told them I loved them before they wheeled me off to the operating room. My last thought before drifting off to sleep was of the beach.

The Beach

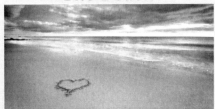

*I sit here and stare straight ahead
It's the beach I'd rather be instead*

*The sand so pure and the sea so blue
Wonderful memories of me and you*

*Sunrise talks
And moonlit walks*

*Your hand in mine
Our promises to stand the test of time*

*With you by my side
I'm confident we can turn the tide*

*It's the picture that hangs on the wall
It reminds me of our trip last Fall*

*As this medicine enters my port
My focus is on that resort*

*Laughing, smiling, the wind in your hair
We'll return again soon, and it will be a wonderful affair*

Approximately ten hours later, I was taken to my hospital room. It was a welcome sight to see my husband, mom and son by my bedside. My son looked apprehensive at first, but I assured him that I was going to be fine, and he gave me a hug. The good news was that the node tested during surgery came back negative which was a tremendous relief. However, the first 24 hours was extremely painful, uncomfortable and exhausting. Because of the type of surgery I had, there were stitches in my chest, as well as my back. I had a total of four drains which needed to be checked and emptied about every two hours, so there was no chance of sleeping. By the third morning, I was more than ready to go home. I got up early, cleaned myself up, and very carefully got dressed. By 10A.M. on January 21st, I was officially released from the hospital. That same night, I had a panic attack when I suddenly couldn't breathe. The pain and pressure in my chest was unbearable. Thankfully, it passed after a few minutes and with my husband and mom by my side I was able to get through it.

Recovery

Going home was a difficult adjustment. A visiting nurse showed me how to properly maintain my drains. I kept a log so that the nurses would be able to determine whether or not they were ready to be removed. I felt a bit like an octopus with multiple limbs. They were uncomfortable and a nuisance, so my goal was to get them taken out as soon as possible. In addition, I kept an accurate recording of when I took pain medication. As sharp as I thought my memory was, the log kept me safe so I wouldn't take too much. Don't misunderstand, I wasn't trying to win any medals for bravery, the first few days it felt good to take a pain pill and fall off to la la land, but I was very aware of the potential dangers too, so I took as little as possible stretched out over time. Besides, it's true what they say about pain medication causing constipation…an unpleasant side effect to everything else going on for sure!

On my second day home, we all agreed I needed to get rid of my "bed head". So my husband and mom took me to my hairdresser (Sharon). It was great to have her wash and blow dry my hair. I felt like a new woman. Sharon had helped several close friends of hers through cancer, and she became a confidant to me as well. I guess it's true that people will open up and tell their hairdressers just about anything because they won't be so judgmental….part hairdresser, part psychiatrist. Although I never took her up on it, she kindly offered to come to the house to do my hair, as well as go shopping for a wig (if it became necessary). In between visits, she would call just to check up on me. She really became a great friend.

Always one to be very independent, I had to learn how to deal with various limitations and rely on others for help. Do to the back latissimus surgery I was swollen, especially under my arms, so my body had to adjust to the muscles being redirected to a new area. An occupational therapist helped me to figure out how best to maneuver around the house which had proven to be a bit challenging. I was unable to raise my arms or lift anything over two pounds and everyday tasks like washing my hair, getting dressed, reaching for anything in cabinets, doing laundry, driving, grocery shopping, etc. were either off limits or I found creative workarounds.

Since lying flat was too difficult, I slept in a recliner for the first few weeks. It made getting up and down bearable. Our family dog slept by my side keeping vigil as if he knew something was off. When washing my hair I would sit on the built-in shower seat, bend forward and flip my head over. This seemed to do the job just fine. Similarly, I would use the same hair flip position when drying my hair (outside of the shower, of course!). If no one was home to help me reach for something in a closet or cabinet, I would use a step stool. Hangers became great tools for lifting clothes out of the closet, and button down shirts were almost a must for several weeks. My family was incredibly helpful too, especially my husband.

He was my rock, juggling everything around the house, the kids, as well as running his own business. While all the focus was on me and my recovery, I was worried about him. We don't have family close by, so we had to rely on each other. In some ways, it made me realize just how much they could do on their own without me. By gosh, and I laugh as I write this, they did know how to make their beds and clean up after themselves!

Slowing down and taking time to heal was hard when I was use to always being on the go, but my body needed time to recover. It constantly let me know if I was pushing things too far. The biggest change in my routine was not being able to exercise and coach my skaters at the rink. My new work out regimen consisted of various stretches given to me by my occupational therapist to do at home; while I relied on other coaches to work with my students in my absence. It would be eight long weeks before I would return to the ice, so I looked forward with anticipation to their updates on how the girls were progressing. Eventually, I would return to both the gym and the rink, apprehensive at first, but it would feel good to get back.

While on the mend, my extended family and friends were

very supportive. They sent books to keep me busy, flowers to brighten my days, soaps and perfumes to make me feel good, cards and texts to offer encouragement, phone calls to lift my spirits, and food to fill my soul. Their outpouring of love was like being wrapped in a blanket. Odd as it may sound, in a positive way, cancer had reconnected me with friends from my past that I hadn't heard from in ages and it truly was wonderful.

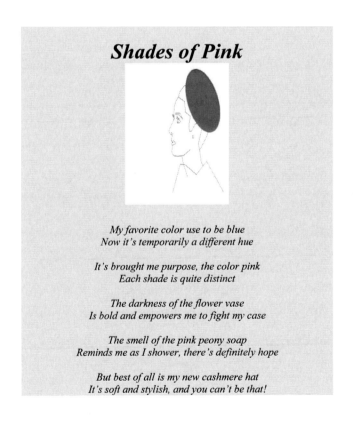

Shades of Pink

My favorite color use to be blue
Now it's temporarily a different hue

It's brought me purpose, the color pink
Each shade is quite distinct

The darkness of the flower vase
Is bold and empowers me to fight my case

The smell of the pink peony soap
Reminds me as I shower, there's definitely hope

But best of all is my new cashmere hat
It's soft and stylish, and you can't be that!

Expect the Unexpected

On February 3rd, as I sat in my office doing computer work, my concentration was interrupted by loud chirping outside my window. When I turned to see what was causing the ruckus, I spotted a red cardinal perched on our water fountain peering back at me. He was no more than six feet away from my window. After a few seconds he flew to a nearby tree, and then came back to the fountain. I stood and went to the window. He stared at me chirping away as if he was trying to tell me something or… warn me. I know that sounds strange, but this was the second time a cardinal had gotten my attention with its relentless chirping. I asked myself, *"Could it be the same cardinal?"* He flew back and forth from the tree to the fountain a few more times before disappearing from my sight.

An hour later, a visiting nurse explained that my back was retaining fluid and it would need to be drained by my doctor. Shortly after her visit, my breast surgeon called with some shocking news regarding my pathology report. First, she confirmed that the cancer had been stage 1. Next, she explained that the tissue removed and sent to the lab for further testing indicated that there had been 3 (not 2) cancerous tumors in my left breast. The fact that there had been a third tumor never detected by the 3-D mammogram, ultrasound or MRI left me stunned. Certainly they were the best tools available to doctors to diagnose breast cancer, but hard to believe that all this technology had missed what had been growing inside of me. Caught completely off guard, I was not prepared for the next part of the conversation.

Once again, the report reconfirmed that the lymph nodes were clear; however, there was concern that there was still a small area (3-4 millimeters) right beneath the surface of the skin with microscopic cancerous cells which meant I would need more surgery to remove more skin and tissue by the site of the initial tumor that I had discovered. Lastly, she mentioned that two of the tumors removed during surgery would be sent out for additional testing, referred to as an Oncotype DX which would further evaluate the oncogene to determine whether or not chemotherapy would be required. We expected the tumors to be tested so that was not a surprise; however, I was dumbfounded and frozen in my chair when she recommended a consultation with a radiologist.

Although it wasn't the first time I broke down, and

certainly not the last, I began to understand just how unpredictable cancer could be. While I knew from the start that radiation and/or chemotherapy could be a part of my treatment, nothing really prepares you for when the doctor actually suggests it could become a reality. Even though her suggestion was precautionary, we decided to wait on a consult until after the second surgery. Our hope was that if she successfully removed the "positive margin" of cells, that radiation might not be necessary.

While we awaited my second surgery, my body had to heal first. When I was given a date of February 27th for my surgery, I sadly realized that once again, I would have to miss out on another significant moment for one of my children. My daughter's synchronized skating team had qualified for the National Synchronized Skating Championship being held in Rhode Island the same weekend of my surgery. My normal patient disposition was just about depleted. I hated that the cancer was all consuming and robbing such special moments from me and my family. I was feeling rather depressed, but then I began to think about others who had been through so much more than me, especially my sister in-law and cousin. Just as I was at my wits end, one of my sisters called and said that she would attend the competition for me. She was a lifesaver when I needed her most!

One morning I looked in the mirror and remembered what someone had said to me, "breast cancer may be the worst year of your life, but once you get through it, it will be behind you, it won't own you forever." They were right. I was a fighter and I would do whatever was necessary to rid my body of this disease.

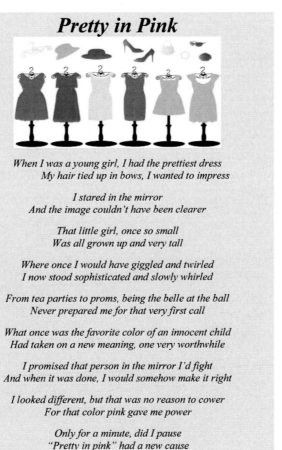

Pretty in Pink

When I was a young girl, I had the prettiest dress
My hair tied up in bows, I wanted to impress

I stared in the mirror
And the image couldn't have been clearer

That little girl, once so small
Was all grown up and very tall

Where once I would have giggled and twirled
I now stood sophisticated and slowly whirled

From tea parties to proms, being the belle at the ball
Never prepared me for that very first call

What once was the favorite color of an innocent child
Had taken on a new meaning, one very worthwhile

I promised that person in the mirror I'd fight
And when it was done, I would somehow make it right

I looked different, but that was no reason to cower
For that color pink gave me power

Only for a minute, did I pause
"Pretty in pink" had a new cause

Symbolism

On the 12th of February, I decided it was best to at least schedule an appointment with a radiologist so that I would be on their calendar post-surgery. I no sooner hung up the phone with the doctor's office when I heard a noise… chirping. As I stood in my kitchen and looked towards the source of the noise, there it was, a cardinal in all its beauty chirping with its fiery crown erect. He was perched on the railing of our deck. As I walked to our sliding glass door, the bird flew to a spot on the deck right in front of me. He looked at me and started chirping again. It was so loud and high pitched, I was captivated by him. This was the third time in three months that a cardinal had caught my attention. *Was it a fluke?* I don't know, but things were about to get a little bit stranger.

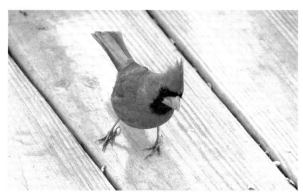

We spent the weekend that followed in the Washington, DC area for a hockey tournament for my son. As my husband drove to DC, I decided to do some internet research on cardinals and dreams about whale sharks. Up until this point, I hadn't mentioned my dream or the reappearance of the cardinals to anyone, including my husband. After checking into the hotel, we decided to relax in our room for a bit. As I sat down on the bed and began to share what had been happening and explaining the research I had been doing, my husband stopped me mid-sentence. He suggested I look at the wall behind me. As I turned, I could not believe my eyes, but there were two framed sketches of cardinals on the wall. While my husband, ever the skeptic, thought it was merely a coincidence and smiled for the first time in weeks; I, on the other hand, was beginning to think otherwise. What were the chances that these cardinal visits and now the pictures were simply a coincidence? I was convinced that these momentary cardinal visits and signs were meant to bring me solace.

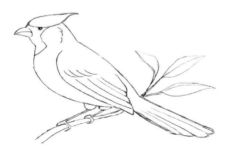

Here is what I learned from my research regarding the red cardinal:

> **Symbolism of the Red Cardinal**
>
> **Red color-** It is meant to get attention, especially in times of grief and depression. Red is a primary color meant to have a powerful presence. For Christians, the color is symbolic of the blood of Christ, as well as, the hope and humanity gained from his resurrection. It is worn by the Cardinals (the highest priests in the Roman Catholic Church) as a sign of steadfast faith.
> **Cycle of 12-** Cardinals are year-round residents. Twelve is considered a powerful cycle in nature as it represents the full spectrum of seasons and the full circle of life. Even their eggs hatch within twelve days.
> **Sound-** The sound, or call, is like "cheer, cheer" to get our attention. It is meant to cheer us up and lead us on an upward journey through the cycle of life.
> **Parenting-** The caring manor of the male may remind us we're not alone and that there is a father above who will always protect and care for us.
> **Health-** A visit from a cardinal could suggest that one's current diet may be injurious to one's health; a sign that we must fight for our health. When the fiery crown rises, it lets us know that we have the strength of spirit within us to win the fight.

If I had read this information prior to these cardinal visits, I would have seriously thought I was consciously projecting the symbolism of these visits onto my situation; however, I honestly had never given the cardinal a second thought (other than it was a beautiful bird), until now. As I tried to digest what I had uncovered, I thought long and hard about the last time I had seen a cardinal, and it hit me. During the time I had lost my pregnancies, there had been a cardinal that appeared outside my office window every day for about a month. I remembered thinking to myself *"what a pretty bird"*. At such a difficult time in our lives, I looked for that beautiful bird every day to cheer myself up. Although I had put it out of my mind, now as I reflected on it, perhaps he was there to comfort me back then. I was convinced that these were not your typical bird sightings. I felt strongly that this bird was purposely coming to my attention at a time of great stress to let me know that I was going to have to fight, and subconsciously, I had a feeling that I would be alright.

After reading the information about the cardinal, my interest was certainly peaked even more about the dream I had had with the whale sharks. They say that dreams are fragments related to life. Here is what I discovered about whale sharks:

Symbolism of the Whale Shark

Image- Their existence in dreams can be influenced by our experiences, beliefs and religion. They are a symbol of strength, spirituality and protection.
Parenting- The whale shark can provide the feeling of a loving mother protecting her child. They represent trust, strength, freedom, safety and love. Since they are associated with peace, serenity and tranquility, their appearance signifies that everything will be okay.
Appearance- They appear when one is facing an overwhelming issue in life. Since whale sharks live underwater they can be seen as our own personal underworld and are viewed as the things we don't want others to know about us or a hidden darkness within us.

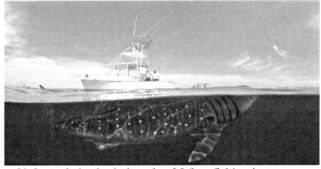
50 foot whale shark dwarfs a 25 foot fishing boat

I remembered when we took our family excursion to swim with the whale sharks that I was in awe of their sheer size (they can grow to the length of a school bus) and strength; yet, as large as these whale sharks were, they were the most harmless gentle creatures. They glided so effortlessly through the ocean, it was beautiful to watch. We had taken some crazy adventures in years past…swimming in the ocean with sharks, barracudas, eels, and sting rays…but this was different, I never felt so much peace swimming with mammals in the ocean then I did on that day. Therefore, it didn't surprise me that if my real-life situation was going to affect my dreams that whale sharks would appear because I would not be afraid. It reminded me of a happy and adventurous time spent with my family.

Weighing the Options

Once again, I found myself in a holding pattern waiting for surgery. Per my doctor's recommendation, I began to do physical therapy. The exercises certainly started to make a difference with increasing my range of motion and improving my level of pain. When February 27th finally rolled around I was eager to get surgery behind me so we could move forward with a long-term plan of action. It was such a small area to pinpoint, like finding a needle in a haystack, all we could do was hope for the best.

A few days later we received a phone call from my breast surgeon with the results of surgery...*no cancerous cells found*. I knew before the doctor said it that this was not the result she had hoped for. The disappointment in her voice echoed through the receiver. In a strange way I found myself feeling more sympathetic for her than me. The whole point of the surgery was to remove lingering cancerous cells, so when they weren't found by the pathologist, I knew it wasn't good, or was it? We held out hope that the earlier pathology report was very conservative and recommended the second surgery when in fact it may not have been necessary. Even my reconstructive doctor who had done countless surgeries with my breast surgeon over the years refused to believe that all the cancer hadn't been removed. It was all so surreal. *Could this really be happening? How much more could be cut from my body?* At this point, it didn't make sense to go back for more surgery. Instead, my doctor recommended a radiologist on staff to review my situation.

Around the same time, I received a phone call from one of my close friends who had been a college classmate. She had had her annual mammogram and they discovered a tumor. This news sent me reeling as I could hear the panic in her voice, and I knew all too well what she was going through. Separated by several States, it crushed me that I couldn't be there in person for her, but just as she had been a rock for me, I vowed to be just as supportive of her. My own personal experience enabled me to provide her with questions to ask her doctors and guide her to various resources for information. Needless to say, we burned up a lot of airtime and text minutes over the next few months. We got through it together.

Prior to meeting with the radiologist, we had a follow up

appointment with my oncologist to review the results of the Onco report. Once again, it was like we were on a combat mission assessing the risks.

First, she explained that the Onco report assigns a number to the tumor on a scale from 1 to 100 in order to determine the risk of cancer recurrence. According to the latest studies, if the tumor falls in the range of 1-18, your risk is considered low; therefore, chemotherapy would not be recommended. A tumor rated greater than 31 is considered high risk requiring chemotherapy; while a tumor rated in between 18 and 31 is considered the intermediate or the "gray" area, where a patient and doctor would need to consider all the facts before determining whether or not to proceed with chemotherapy. Studies claimed that approximately 50% of patients who fall into the low risk category still have a 10% chance of **recurrence elsewhere in the body** (i.e. lymph nodes, liver, bone) even with stage 1 cancer. Since my tumors fell into the low risk category, I would **not need** chemotherapy. This was a huge relief; however, the plan was to immediately start me on a hormone therapy drug (Tamoxifen) to help reduce the risk of recurrence as much as possible.

As long as I was considered pre-menopausal I would be on

Tamoxifen for the next five years. If I began menopause during that time, they would switch my medication to a different aromatase inhibitor (aka. hormone therapy drug). Depending on the outcome of studies currently in progress, the medication could be extended to 10 years, but that would be determined at a much later date. In the meantime, I would pray every day that this tiny white pill would ward off the enemy from raising its ugly head again.

My breast surgeon joined us for the next part of the discussion in regards to radiation. The reason to radiate the area in question (where the small margin of cells were identified) was to minimize the chance of **local recurrence of breast cancer at the same site**. The consensus being that radiation would help to reduce the risk to single digits. Both doctors felt that without it, the chance of local recurrence could increase as much as 20%.

If I elected not to radiate the area, they would continue to monitor me closely with physical exams and MRIs every 6 months the first year, then once a year for 3 years. This was a lot to digest. It was almost like being diagnosed all over again. The positives were: I had stage 1 breast cancer, low grade tumors less than 2cm in size, clear nodes, a non-aggressive type cancer, a negative BRCA test, and low Onco scores. In addition, we weren't necessarily convinced that the doctor hadn't removed the positive margin of microscopic cells. Perhaps the pathology lab missed something. My brain felt like a mouse on an exercise wheel, running... running the statistics over and over again in my head. I was so confused about what to do, it was unnerving.

To make matters worse, when I left my doctors' office I got a distraught phone call from my college friend whose biopsy confirmed she had breast cancer. Sadly, my circle of eight hadn't been spared. This was crazy...I wanted to scream, but instead, I cried. I cried for my friend, and I cried because I was scared to make the wrong choice (*radiate or not radiate*).

Despite being surrounded by an amazing support group of family and friends, I realized just how isolating cancer could be. Alone with my own thoughts, fears and decisions, it could be paralyzing at times. Ironically, around this time, a friend texted me a message that helped to pull me out of my funk...

Even when you're hurting find a way to keep going. A strong woman never gives up!

Rainbows

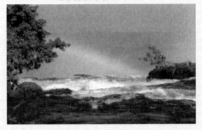

Stay strong, because a positive attitude will make things clearer. Look to brighter skies ahead and you'll find beauty in the mirror.

Stay strong, because things will get better. It might be stormy now, but the rain can't last forever.

Stay strong, because dancing in the rain can be fun. And when the storm passes you'll find solace by the sun.

Stay strong, because despite the clouds that may darken your way, look for the rainbow in every day

Power of Prayer

On the morning of my appointment with the radiologist, I sat in my kitchen enjoying a cup of coffee. I was reviewing my notes from my last doctor's appointment and was contemplating what questions to ask this new doctor I was about to meet. Out of the corner of my eye, something moved and caught my attention. My cardinal was back to pay me a visit. He landed atop a table on our deck looking in the window at me. Unlike previous visits, he wasn't chirping, just looking at me. I was caught in a trance with this bird. Although it was Friday the 13th (March), superstitions aside, his presence calmed me and boosted my confidence that I would somehow make the right decision.

The radiologist was a lovely doctor who patiently walked me through a number of statistics and the recommended treatment. For a patient with invasive breast cancer, stage 1, negative lymph nodes, tumors less than 5 cm with "close" margins (a millimeter of microscopic cancer cells), the recommendation was to consider radiation therapy every day for six weeks. Yet, the big question mark even among the hospital staff was whether or not those cells or "close" margin still existed. The doctor suggested that I take about a week to decide what I wanted to do.

Over the weekend we went to church. I said a prayer for our family and asked God for guidance as I stood at this crossroad. This was the second most important decision of my life and I needed his help. I felt very strongly that I was going to be fine even without radiation. And, if by chance something did recur later on in life, we would deal with it just as we had over the last year. As mass began, the choir opened with a song…"*These Alone Are Enough*". The song spoke to me and I was no longer afraid. I had offered up grace and was resolute in my decision. I felt the weight of the world lift off my shoulders. For the first time in five months, I was truly at peace, and it was liberating.

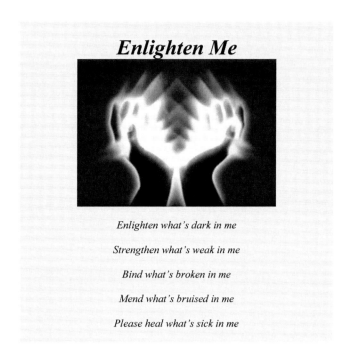

Enlighten what's dark in me

Strengthen what's weak in me

Bind what's broken in me

Mend what's bruised in me

Please heal what's sick in me

One Two Punch

When the radiologist called the following week, and I shared my decision not to pursue radiation, she said, "I think you made the best decision for you." She wished me a long healthy life and hoped that if our paths crossed again that it would be under much better circumstances. It felt good not to be questioned, but rather her affirmation was exactly what I needed to start the healing process. I don't know why, it may sound crazy, but I felt like I had just won the match of my life.

As I entered my home office to write in my journal, I looked out the window, there was my cardinal flying back and forth between the fountain and a birdfeeder. It was almost like he was doing a dance between the two objects. I like to think of it as a victory dance.

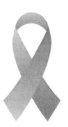

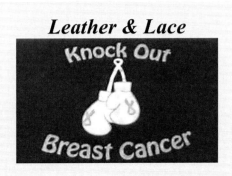

*I looked cancer in the face
It may be a tough fight
But my gloves are leather and lace*

*I looked cancer in the face
I will be a force to contend with
As I move around the ring with grace*

*I looked cancer in the face
I gave it a one-two punch
Now there's not a trace*

*I looked cancer in the face
I will work tirelessly to educate women
Against the clock, we will race*

*I looked cancer in the face
Put up your dukes and join the match
Please don't stop fighting, till it's finally erased*

In a Fog

"Mom, I just told you five minutes ago," my son would say to me. *"Oh yeah, that's right. Sorry!"* would be my standard reply. I was cognizant of the fact that I was struggling to remember the simplest things...a conversation, a word I had used a thousand times or a story from my past. We joked about mom getting old and ignored it, but after some time passed I needed to know what was happening to me. Back to doing some research on-line, I found my answer. Although I didn't need to have chemotherapy and decided to forego radiation, I began to experience something called "mind fog" or "chemo brain". It was frustrating, especially since for almost twenty years of my adult life I had managed project managers in the telecom industry where attention to detail was crucial. Pulling things out of my memory bank had never been an issue for me. Now there were days where remembering where I put my glasses was a challenge. I asked my sister-in-law if she was experiencing the same thing. As a teacher, she struggled as well trying to relay lesson plans and remember facts she had been teaching for years.

What I learned was that this was a known side effect from treatments, such as: chemotherapy, radiation, and anesthesia (usually much more temporary). The more treatments one had, the longer they could potentially experience this issue. It also could be brought on by hormonal changes and stress. While my sister-in-law's situation was probably do to the chemo and surgeries, I believe mine was related to the stress, surgeries, as well as hormonal changes do to Tamoxifen. I guess I could only hope that this issue wouldn't last for the next five years or I'd be filling journals with notes to be able to recall events and conversations for a long time!

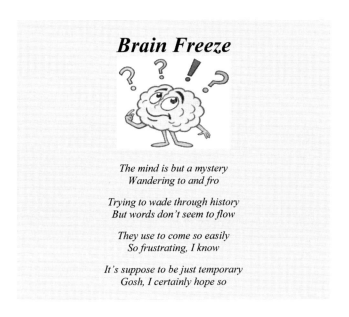

Brain Freeze

The mind is but a mystery
Wandering to and fro

Trying to wade through history
But words don't seem to flow

They use to come so easily
So frustrating, I know

It's suppose to be just temporary
Gosh, I certainly hope so

Healing

The next six months would be consumed with more doctor visits and surgery to fill and eventually swap the tissue expanders for implants and to complete reconstructing the aesthetics of the breasts.

Stitches

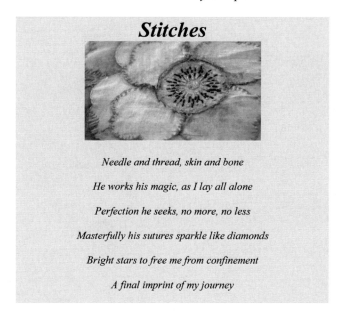

Needle and thread, skin and bone

He works his magic, as I lay all alone

Perfection he seeks, no more, no less

Masterfully his sutures sparkle like diamonds

Bright stars to free me from confinement

A final imprint of my journey

As my body was healing, I felt my mind needed to heal as well, so I took a few classes (i.e. nutrition, art, yoga & meditation) with other survivors. Having been a person who has exercised for years, I knew yoga & meditation were going to be a challenge. Any exercise that didn't produce sweat just didn't seem to cut it for me. As I stood in a circle of other women, breathing in and exhaling out, my mind raced all about consumed with where I needed to go next versus relaxing and holding various poses. But, I have to admit, when we sat on the floor to begin our meditation, I managed to relax myself just enough to where I felt myself floating among clouds. The instructor's voice was quite soothing. Just as I was about to fall deeper, someone's phone rang, snapping me back to reality. As I peered out of one eye, everyone else appeared so Zen-like. They were able to ignore the background noise. Sadly, I crept from class as the spell had been broken, yet elated that I had tried it.

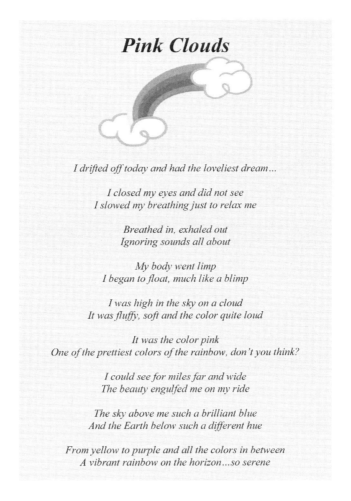

Pink Clouds

I drifted off today and had the loveliest dream...

*I closed my eyes and did not see
I slowed my breathing just to relax me*

*Breathed in, exhaled out
Ignoring sounds all about*

*My body went limp
I began to float, much like a blimp*

*I was high in the sky on a cloud
It was fluffy, soft and the color quite loud*

*It was the color pink
One of the prettiest colors of the rainbow, don't you think?*

*I could see for miles far and wide
The beauty engulfed me on my ride*

*The sky above me such a brilliant blue
And the Earth below such a different hue*

*From yellow to purple and all the colors in between
A vibrant rainbow on the horizon...so serene*

Healing...doesn't mean the damage never existed. It means the damage no longer control our lives.

The Finish Line

Not too long before my diagnosis I ran the Susan G. Komen Race for the Cure in Philadelphia with my daughter 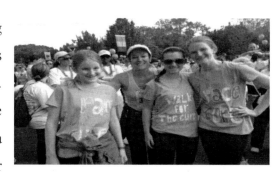 and friends. To witness the thousands of women, men and children who turn out to volunteer, walk or run the race, is nothing short of amazing. The city was a sea of pink. It was emotional to say the least. We vowed to do the race every year as a tradition. Sadly, that plan was temporarily placed on hold when I found myself in the midst of my own fight. However, I'm proud to say that in September, I ran a mile for the first time in nine months. It felt a bit awkward, but nothing that a good sports bra couldn't fix! As I continue to work on building my stamina, I look forward to running in the next race in honor of my family and friends touched by this disease.

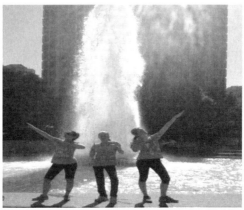
My daughter and friends striking their warrior pose.

On October 6, 2015, I had my last visit with my plastic surgeon. His work was done… masterpiece complete! Strangely enough, it was a bittersweet feeling. While I was relieved to be moving on with one less doctor to visit, I was a little sad that these extraordinary people (the doctor, nurses, and staff) would not be in my life anymore. In the midst of our crisis, it seemed like it would take forever to be done with, but now, almost in a blink of an eye, it was over. With a hug and a good-bye, I had "graduated"…one step closer to the finish line. The **finish line…** W*here or when exactly would I cross it? Would it be the one year anniversary of my diagnosis? Would it be my next MRI? Or five to ten years from now when I finished hormone therapy?* The allusive finish line seemed almost within reach, yet just far enough out of grasp to make me wonder...*what if?* A lingering thought that sometimes snuck in, but I quickly pushed it aside, to focus on the positives and the here and now. Besides, there would be on-going visits with my breast surgeon and oncologist over the coming months and years, so I felt strongly that the worst was now behind me...in my rearview mirror, becoming more and more distant with each passing curve in the road.

A year had passed, Fall had returned, the leaves were turning a magnificent color, and it felt good to open the windows and let the cool air in. I was alive and it was exhilarating. When I returned home from my doctor's appointment I sat down at my desk to write. As I turned to look outside to gather my thoughts, not one, but two cardinals landed on the fountain outside of my window. It was the first time I had seen one since March, the day of my radiologist appointment. They were taking turns splashing around as if they were having a party. My cardinal had brought a friend to celebrate! Trying not to scare them away, I carefully grabbed my phone and snapped some pictures. I wanted proof to show my husband and a photo that would last a lifetime. This bird had become a token of love, faith and hope. It had appeared at my darkest hour giving me strength and courage, and again on one of my happiest days giving me peace of mind and making me smile.

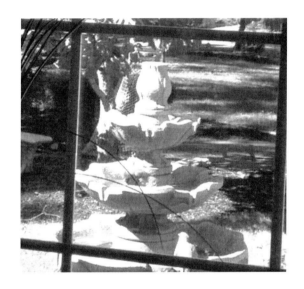

So go outside and look to the trees, for that's where the little red bird will be. Do not fear an angel will appear to let you know your loved one is near.

Reflection

There was a time in May when I started to question the direction of this book. Would it become a book? Would anyone be interested in reading it? Did I really have something to say that mattered? Or had this urge to write just been therapeutic to help me through my own personal strife? I felt that I was led to my answer simply by a trip to the local book store.

One day while I was out running errands, my husband asked me to pick him up a book. As I entered the book store, out of the corner of my eye, a bright color caught my attention. The book had a vivid blue cover, but it was the red that really peeked my interest. My first thought was that it was a cardinal, but at a closer glance I could see it was a brilliant red leaf on a bare tree with the brightest blue sky and fluffiest clouds for a backdrop. The name of the book was When God Winks at You by Squire Rushnell. The idea expressed in the book is that sometimes events occur in our lives that on the surface may appear to be coincidences, but are truly messages – or *godwinks* - from God meant to bring us some level of comfort. Messages to let you know He's there and He's listening. The author, who had been an executive at one time with ABC, shared his story of how difficult it had been to get published. Even with his media connections, he didn't give up. Eight years it took him, but his story finally went to print. Of the thousands of books in the store that day, why was I drawn to this particular book? Was this a *godwink* for me...a message that I should continue with my own book? It certainly re-energized me and reminded me why I started to write to begin with. It wasn't about fame, fortune or notoriety, that's for sure! I had written and self-published two children's books prior to this one, so I knew what I was getting myself in to. The difference with this book was that it was non-fiction, a true story based on real-life circumstances. I have absolutely no medical training in my background; however, if I could somehow help, even one person through this daunting process, by sharing my own personal experience and lessons learned, than I achieved success. Needless to say, I bought the book!

As I left the book store that day, a sun shower was passing by. Steam was rising from the pavement as the rain cooled the tar from the blistering heat of the sun. I stopped and smelled the rain, really smelled the rain. *Have you ever smelled the rain?* It definitely has a very distinct smell. I looked to the sky and let the rain wash over me. It felt cool and crisp on my warm skin. As people scurried to their cars, I looked down at a puddle and saw my reflection.

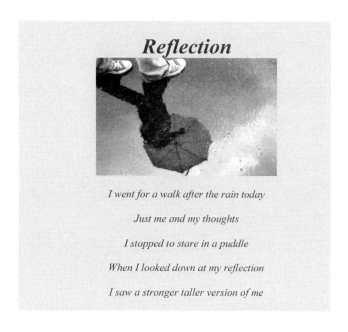

Reflection

I went for a walk after the rain today

Just me and my thoughts

I stopped to stare in a puddle

When I looked down at my reflection

I saw a stronger taller version of me

When God Winks at You was such an inspirational story that I started to keep track of some of my own *"godwinks"* along the way. Just like anybody else, I have good days and bad days, but I find that when I reflect on these scenarios over the past months, they make me smile.

When we met with the first breast surgeon for a consultation she touched my husband's shoulder and looked into his eyes and said, "Everything will be okay." And she hugged me when I stood up whispering, "He really loves you." It was a simple, yet extremely warm gesture. With a name that sounded like "fantastic", she was fantastic! Although our insurance did not enable me to see her again, I have since referred friends to her.

Before I was taken into the operating room my breast surgeon and reconstructive doctors stopped by to review my surgery. Upon their departure my mom began to cry, without hesitation, my breast surgeon walked over and gave her a hug. It was a simple act of kindness that I will never forget.

Towards the end of January, I had my first follow up appointment with my reconstructive doctor. The waiting room was packed on this particular visit so I found two open seats for my husband and I among three other women. One lady sat down and whispered to the group of us, "Have you seen the bathroom here ladies?" We all smiled and said, "Yes." She continued, "I think I'm going to take pictures next time. I've never seen such a beautiful bathroom in a doctor's office!" We all laughed. It was a great ice breaker and broke the deafening silence in the room. We immediately struck up a conversation. All four of us were at different stages with our treatment. One lady mentioned that she was in her 30's with two young children at home. She had a very similar diagnosis as me, had had the same surgery a few weeks prior to me, and had just learned the day before she would not need chemo. The next lady, who seemed pleasantly plump, was approximately in her late 60's. I got the impression she was newly diagnosed and was there for a consultation. However, as she wiggled in her seat, she did say, "At my age and size I won't be wearing any bikinis to the beach, so I'm not sure why I'm here!" Again, we all laughed, but I thought to myself...how brave of her to be considering no reconstruction as an option. The third woman had been diagnosed for the second time in ten years and had just finished chemo. She was 60 and stunning. If she hadn't mentioned that she bought her latest wig at a local flea market, I would have never been the wiser. Having spent $1500 on a wig the first time she went through chemo, she was thrilled to brag about her flea market find at $50, especially since co-workers and acquaintances kept asking who her hair stylist was! She claimed that it was such a big hit, she went back and bought it in other colors so she could "really throw them for a loop!" My stitches and chest hurt, but it still felt good to laugh. Lastly, this sweet woman went on to share with us that she had tried using olive oil on her scalp because she had read that it promoted hair re-growth. Of course, we were all curious to know if she thought it worked, she burst out laughing and said that it dripped into her eyes and burned so much that she washed it right out. She added, "Next time I think I'll try extra virgin olive oil!" She had us laughing so much I was crying. It felt good to laugh with these women who understood what I was going through. Laughter was good medicine to momentarily take my mind off the physical pain. When the nurse called my name I excused myself and said it was time to go get my Botox treatment. They laughed and wished me luck!

Around March I decided to create a Facebook page for family, friends and acquaintances who had endured breast cancer themselves or knew someone who had battled the disease. I wanted it to be a safe place for people to share tips and/or poetry with one another. As I began to post information, I was blessed in return by reconnecting with old childhood friends who had fought their own battles and were willing to share their stories. It became a source of comfort for me.

On vacation in Florida, an elderly woman approached me in the grocery store on Easter and said, "I use to look as good as you once." I laughed and thought to myself...must be the dress! Two days later a woman walked up to me in the pool and said, "You look great in that bathing suit." Never in my life had a complete stranger complimented my appearance, let alone two in the same week! This was shortly after I had started the expansion process and was feeling a bit self-conscientious. I found their timing humorous and thought...perhaps 50 won't be so bad after all!

One afternoon I arrived home from seeing my reconstructive doctor for the second and final expansion. I decided to check the mailbox. When I opened the box and pulled out the mail, I suddenly found myself wet all down the front of my pants. For some reason there was water leaking from a package. As I investigated it further, I noticed the package was from a family friend in Ireland. When I showed the package to my husband, he said, "Oh no, it must have broke." "What broke?" I asked. I had no idea we were expecting something. As he opened the package he explained that his friend had bought holy water on a trip to Fatima (in Portugal) and shipped it when he got home to Ireland. My husband looked at me, smiled and said, "Consider yourself blessed!" That bottle of holy water had traveled all that way without breaking until I pulled it out of our mailbox. Was it a coincidence or godwink?

In July, I had the opportunity to meet up with a very dear friend at the beach. We have been friends since middle school. Although miles have separated us since college, we've always stayed in touch. She was truly an amazing friend through my entire ordeal. As we sat down on the beach, I heard a twin engine plane over head. The sign behind it was an advertisement for my hospital with a question that read, "Have you applied your sunblock?" Really?! First time at the beach all summer and that's the first sign I see. I had to laugh. As my friend and I continued to exchange pleasantries, she told me about a friend she had lost earlier in the year to cancer and that she had been drawn to cardinals throughout her treatment. Up until this day, I had never shared anything about my cardinal visits with anyone other than my husband. I found it *reassuring that this other woman had found peace with her cardinal visits as well. It inspired my friend's boyfriend to write a song titled "Soaring High" which he sang for me that night. It was absolutely beautiful and warmed my heart.*

To someone else, I suppose each of these incidences could be referred to as acts of human kindness or simply coincidences, but I truly feel blessed to have had these experiences and will continue to refer to them as my *godwinks*.

Live Love Laugh

As I was shopping (yes, I like to shop!) for college supplies for my daughter, a sign with the saying Live Love Laugh caught my attention and caused me to pause…it had been almost a year since my initial diagnosis. My daughter had successfully finished her first year at college, my son had won the opportunity to attend hockey camp in Canada, and with the support of my family, friends and top notch doctors, I survived breast cancer. No, I did not experience an epiphany. I have continued to live my life as I always have, accept…I have made a conscientious effort to try desperately not to sweat the small stuff and take more time to appreciate life's little wonders. I suppose like most people who have a medical scare it makes you stop, evaluate things, and really appreciate life and the people in it.

Three simple words that hold so much depth...***Live Love Laugh.*** Ask yourself, do you really "live" your life to the fullest? Take advantage of all that life has to offer? Do you love fully with all your heart? Do you embrace the good, as well as the bad? Do you really laugh? They say that laughter is good for the soul. I'm sure we've all seen these words printed on cards, pictures and various forms of artwork, but never have they really had such an impact on me until now.

To Live: I like to think that I have really lived my life without regrets. In my twenties, I wanted to be independent, pursue my career and travel the world. In my thirties, it was about finding balance between building a life with my husband and family, and juggling a demanding position at work. In my forties, I knew who I was (confident in my beliefs and values) and focused on family and a close-knit group of trusted friends. As I've begun the next decade of my life, I fully embrace it and all that it has to offer. Yes, it started out with a major bump (or lump) in the road, but that's behind me now and I'm ready and excited for the future. A future that I am truly blessed to have after such a scary time. I realize now more than ever that you shouldn't wait to do things because the timing may never be perfect. You just have to go for it. And every day I try to look for my own "rainbow" even if there isn't one in the sky. Sometimes I put on my favorite jewelry on just to make me smile, to add a little "bling" to my day. As they say, you can't dwell on the past and you never know what tomorrow may bring, so grab hold of the present because today is a gift and you might as well enjoy it!

To Love: About a week after we shared my diagnosis with our children, I was cleaning my son's room. As I lifted a pile of books on his desk I noticed some pages with hand-written notes. At the top of the very first page it read: *Why did mom get cancer?* The pages that followed were filled with facts my son had diligently researched on the internet. It broke my heart that my twelve year old son was consumed by his mom's illness rather than school, sports and friends. Yet, it made me smile to know he cared so much and, like his dad, wanted to know everything he could to try and make the situation better. I truly was blessed with an amazing family. I never knew I could love my husband any more than I already did, but I do believe our love and appreciation for one another grew profoundly during this time.

To Laugh: I think laughter is like medicine, it's good for the sole and one's health. We all experience good days and bad days, it's just a part of life, but I really try to focus more energy on the positive and staying upbeat. No one else can make you happy, but you, it starts from within. I have found that when you're happy and smiling, more often than not, people around you respond. I do believe that happiness is contagious and if you're hanging around someone who's always focused on the sour grapes, then, perhaps it's time to make some adjustments. Life's too short to let outside influences sap all the positive energy out of a room, a day, or particular situation. There were several occasions over the last few months where certain scenarios or comments made me laugh or smile. Here are just a few I thought I'd share:

An acquaintance who heard about my illness said to me, "I'm sorry to hear what you're going through, but you don't look sick." I smiled because I know they meant this in a positive way, but I thought, "What am I suppose to look like?

What does cancer look like?" Naively, I once thought that all breast cancer patients either lost their hair to chemo or, at a minimum, went through radiation. So maybe that's what they were really thinking...she doesn't look sick because she hasn't lost her hair. It really opened my eyes to the fact that you never know what burden someone may be carrying.

The first day I attempted to drive (post-surgery), I got in the car and turned on the radio. The first song I heard was Warrior by Demi Lovato, immediately followed by Fight Song, by Rachel Platten. I couldn't think of two more appropriate songs given my personal circumstances. My kids will be the first to tell you that I maintain a certain low volume when driving, but on this day, I threw caution to the wind. Blasting those tunes lifted my spirits for sure!

One afternoon I had an appointment with my oncologist. We were there to discuss hormone therapy treatment. When she started down the list of potential side-effects, I felt like I was watching one of those TV infomercials. My husband and I burst out laughing when she mentioned the fact that the prescription drug I would be taking could increase fertility. What?! At 50, getting pregnant was the last thing on my mind. Someone in a science lab sure had a sense of humor...let's develop a drug to avert cancer from reoccurring, but it may have about fifteen side-effects (i.e. hot flashes, mood swings, depression, nausea, weight gain, increased fertility). It sounded like five years of torture! I don't mean to sound unappreciative of the fact that one tiny pill a day could be a lifesaver, but my initial reaction was...only a guy would have come up with this one! Now every morning I dutifully take my pill and pray to remain cancer-free and pregnant-free!!

During the summer we took a vacation to Canada. Our first stop was Niagara Falls, one of the natural wonders of the world. We had the opportunity the first night of our trip to see it lit up. It was a spectrum of colors, like a rainbow. It was magnificent. The next afternoon we saw it again. I was awestruck by its sheer size and strength. Once again, I didn't have to look too far for my rainbow on this particular day. As a tour boat approached the Falls, far below my perch high up on a cliff, I could see a vibrant rainbow above the boat. It truly was a spectacular site.

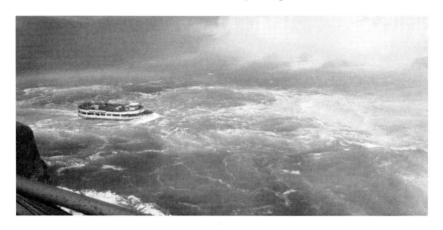

 In mid-August, my husband was on a mission to keep us awake one night to watch for a meteor shower. He and my daughter watched from our deck as my son and I kept vigil from our bedroom windows. I have to say it was worth the wait. Thanks to a brilliant moon that night, the sky was clear and the meteor shower did not disappoint. We could hear neighbors howling "ooh" and "ah" every time a meteor went zipping across. It was a natural firework display in the sky... simply incredible!

Star Struck

I marvel at the moon so bright
Nature's bulb has turned on the light

Night has summoned all God's creatures to thrive
A symphony of sounds have come alive

A plethora of diamonds have suddenly arisen
Producing a constellation that glistens

Fireworks falling into the dark abyss
They ignite a spark like a first kiss

Whizzing at lightning speed across the night sky
Some too fast for the human eye

Made a wish just in case
Before it's extinguished without a trace

One night in October, I decided to have a "bra burning" party in my backyard to destroy the mastectomy bras and camisoles I wore post-surgery. I also wrote a letter to my cancer. My husband lit our fire pit and I threw them in one at a time releasing all the anger, guilt and fear into the flames. When we were done, we made s'mores and toasted with a glass of wine. I couldn't think of a better way to celebrate being cancer-free, especially during breast cancer awareness month.

On the Bright Side

It was a very long stressful year. There were times when we felt we took two steps forward, only to take three steps backward. Cancer tested every ounce of patience within me, but didn't kill my spirit or determination. With a lot of hope, faith in my doctors and God, and love from family and friends, I made it through this past year. My scars tell my story of survival. They represent the fact that I showed up for the fight and didn't run from it. I know in time, my physical pain, as well as my scars, will fade as has my mental anguish. More importantly, and my eyes well up with tears as I write this, I am a… **survivor**. My cancer scare certainly gave me reason to pause. As the seasons changed, so did I; I thank God every day for waking up and giving me a chance to really appreciate the people in my life and the beauty all around me.

The seasons have changed, and so have I...

Winter brought snow from the sky,
It reminded me to soar high

Spring sprung showers,
I smelled the beautiful flowers

Summer warmed the touch of my skin,
The taste of the salty air made me glow within

Fall changed the colors to a vibrant hue
The birds chirped loudly getting ready to take their cue

... I've listened, smelled, touched, and saw the most beautiful things this past year.

As life has resumed to a sense of normalcy, I feel I've come to another crossroads. I can choose to move forward and never look back or somehow use the knowledge I gained from this last year to help others. For some survivors sometimes it's just too painful to dwell on everything they've been through which I can completely understand and respect that position. Personally, I plan to become a more active participant in my community as a patient advocate. Writing this book was cathartic and seemed to be an appropriate start in that direction.

If I don't use my experience to help others, then I feel the experience was wasted on me. I intend to focus on volunteering my time to organizations whose funding goes towards researching a cure as well as promoting early detection.

For me, the pink ribbon has become more than a symbol for breast cancer awareness, it's become a sign of hope, strength and courage for the women diagnosed each year. It's the quintessential female color that feels nurturing and provides hope for a cure. While it was not a "club" I actively sought to join, being a breast cancer survivor has really given me purpose to want to help others. I had this bad thing happen to me, now I want to make something good come out of it.

Think Pink

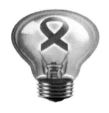

The color pink makes me think...

Pink sand between my toes
Pink bubblegum sweet as cherry
Pink cotton candy at a carnival
Pink dress for a party
Pink scarf to keep warm
Pink hat to be stylish
Pink lipstick to stand out
Pink ribbon as a sign of hope
Pink feather to be a warrior

...Pink is cool

In Honor Of

First and foremost, I would like to acknowledge my sister-in-law Tracy. While fighting her own courageous battle, she truly inspired me and her own family. Despite dealing with her own set of complications, she was always there for my husband and I, offering guidance as well as moral support. I watched with admiration as she was an amazing role model, especially for her children through such adversity.

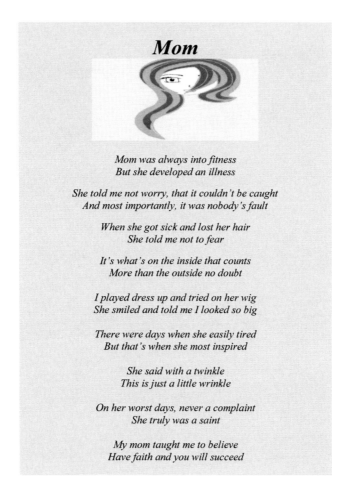

Mom

*Mom was always into fitness
But she developed an illness*

*She told me not worry, that it couldn't be caught
And most importantly, it was nobody's fault*

*When she got sick and lost her hair
She told me not to fear*

*It's what's on the inside that counts
More than the outside no doubt*

*I played dress up and tried on her wig
She smiled and told me I looked so big*

*There were days when she easily tired
But that's when she most inspired*

*She said with a twinkle
This is just a little wrinkle*

*On her worst days, never a complaint
She truly was a saint*

*My mom taught me to believe
Have faith and you will succeed*

Secondly, I would like to mention my dear friend Judy, who aside from dealing with her own personal medical issues was a huge champion of mine. She shared a story with me about her grandmother's battle with breast cancer. Sadly, she passed before Judy was able to develop a relationship with her, but her brave fight was not in vain.

Grandmother

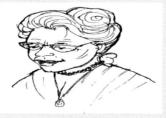

I have a picture of grandma and me
Wrapped in a blanket being bounced on her knee

She was a very strong woman
And her name was simply Susan

Her eyes were warm and gentle
And a voice so soft and peaceful

She sang to me sweet lullabies
To hush my newborn cries

My grandma was one who led the way
A pillar of strength and dignity

She waged a war with a mighty force
Determined to stay the course

Our relationship was rather fleeting
But my love for her ever-lasting

I think of her with much gratitude
And I'll continue to fight with her fortitude

As she is now deceased
May she always rest in peace

I feel in my soul that that cardinal was sent as a messenger from God to watch over me. I miss seeing him, but I like to think he's flown off to help someone else in need. And I truly believe that my father who passed from our world some nineteen years ago was with me during my dream about the whale sharks and those cardinal visits as a way to let me know that he would be there for me when I needed him the most. As a young girl he taught me to be both mentally as well as physically tough through hard work, determination and perseverance. If I stumbled or fell down, he encouraged me to get back up and try again. Quitting was not an option. He had, and still has, a huge influence on my fighting spirit. There's not a day that goes by that I don't think of him, but I felt his presence quite a bit throughout my journey.

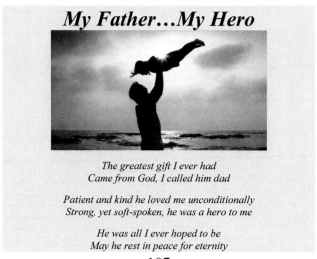

My Father...My Hero

The greatest gift I ever had
Came from God, I called him dad

Patient and kind he loved me unconditionally
Strong, yet soft-spoken, he was a hero to me

He was all I ever hoped to be
May he rest in peace for eternity

And lastly, I couldn't imagine ending my story without paying a special tribute to all the women (or warriors) who have courageously fought their own battle with breast cancer paving the way for better medical tests and furthering the advancement of treatment.

Warrior

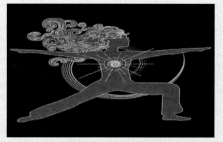

You are strong
even at your weakest

You are powerful
when you feel helpless

You are fearless
when circumstances are scary

You are a survivor
when the battle gets difficult, don't give up

You are a warrior
your strength, power, & courage will win the war

Concluding Thoughts

Life can sometimes throw you a curve ball when you least expect it and put you on a path that you never thought you would walk...

It's true; I never for a second would have thought that I would be diagnosed with breast cancer. For ten years, I faithfully had my annual mammograms and while I was always a bit apprehensive about them, I never really thought it was possible that I could potentially be diagnosed. I suppose naiveté was bliss. Since it didn't run in my family, I thought I was safe.

Distraught with fear, a beacon of light renewed my faith in God, love, and gave me hope that everything would be alright. I'll never question it, but it was just a feeling that I had inside. Those momentary visits from a little red cardinal ignited a spirit to fight and to be strong through the most difficult time of my life.

Soar High

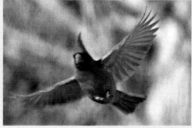

Little red bird
Guiding me to find the right words

You came to me
And set me free

You lifted my burden
Time to help someone else who's hurting

So fly away, fly away
No need to stay

If ever I should need you near
I'll look to heaven and wait for your cheer

Soar high to the sky my beacon of light
Sadly, I'll wave good-bye…as you fly out of sight

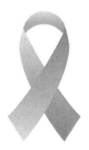

All-Star Team

My story would not be complete without acknowledging and thanking, what I endearingly refer to as, my "all-star" team.

Starting with my medical team, some of who I interacted with only briefly (Dr. Dershem, Dr. Piccoli, Dr. Fantazzio, Dr. Liao, Dr. Hughes, Dr. Waldron, Genetic Counselor Shirley Yao, Nurse Practitioner Helen Nichter) and Nurse Navigator Angela Frantz who patiently guided me through this daunting process. To my breast surgeon (Dr. Brill) who was always willing to take the time to share her medical expertise and offer advice. I never felt rushed as she would call with updates via the phone or sit with us and very carefully explain results. She was (and is) a true patient advocate. To my oncologist (Dr. Grana) who was always very thorough in explaining various tests and my next steps. To my plastic surgeon (Dr. Copit) who took as much pride in his work as Picasso did with his art. And lastly, Margaret Papa, my physical therapist, whose exercises got me moving quickly and whose delicate (yet strong) hands relieved my pain with the most amazing massages.

When a person is diagnosed with breast cancer they spend a lot of time in medical offices. The secretaries, medical assistants, nurses, therapists, as well as the doctors become almost like extended family for a short period of time…they have a vested interest in your health and well being. During my own journey, I got a brief glimpse into some of their lives. I learned that most had been touched by breast cancer in their own families…either a mother, wife, sister, cousin, friend, or even themselves. Perhaps that was the driving force behind why some had pursued their specific occupation…so they could make a difference. Whatever the reason, their willingness to share their own stories was admirable. I couldn't have asked for a better team to be on my side!

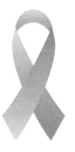

Caregiver

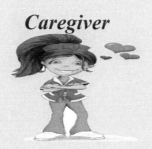

Caregivers come from all walks of life
Miracle workers to help with our strife

They open their hearts, devoting their care
To patients and loved ones who have a scare

To nurture and heal is a tremendous calling
To catch us when we're falling

A selfless gift like no other
Aiding a friend, sister, wife or mother

For these guardians that walk among us
Earn their wings on a daily basis

Sometimes it's the little things people naturally do
That makes our lives brighter and happier too

It might be a kind helping hand
Or simply a whisper, "I understand"

A hug, a thank you, the warmth of a smile
Can certainly make it all worthwhile

For life is a precious gift
So be sure to celebrate the people in it

Next, to my mom (Mary Nowak, RN) who listened, offered advice and kept vigil with my husband during the most difficult time of this journey...I love you and thank you from the bottom of my heart for being there for me.

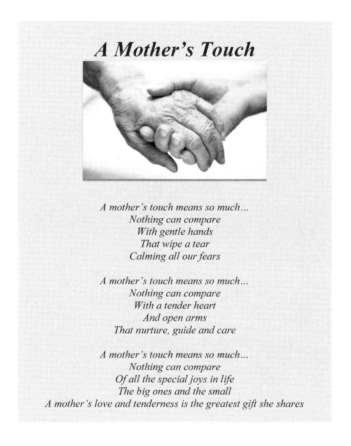

A Mother's Touch

A mother's touch means so much...
Nothing can compare
With gentle hands
That wipe a tear
Calming all our fears

A mother's touch means so much...
Nothing can compare
With a tender heart
And open arms
That nurture, guide and care

A mother's touch means so much...
Nothing can compare
Of all the special joys in life
The big ones and the small
A mother's love and tenderness is the greatest gift she shares

I also have to give a huge shout out to my extended family and friends. To my sisters, brother and my husband's family for constantly offering their help, love, prayers and support.

To my dear friends whose phone calls, text messages, and emails picked me up when I was down. A special thanks to Jill, who took it upon herself to coordinate the delivery of various gifts with other friends over a series of weeks. The outpouring of love brightened my spirits and filled my family's belly! And to Kimberly and her daughters, whose delicious homemade chicken soup warmed my soul...it was the gift that kept on giving!

Dear Friend, My Sister

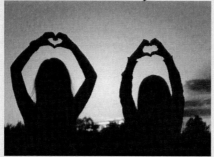

I am blessed to call you sister.
Your honesty is sincere.
You don't judge, but offer patience & understanding.
When I am weak, you give me strength & encouragement.
We've laughed until we've cried, and cried until our cheeks hurt.
We celebrate each other's joys and mourn our sorrows.
Only a true friend can be called sister, and a sister a friend.
One is a gift at birth, and the other is picked like a beautiful flower that grows & blossoms.
I am especially honored to call you friend.

To two complete strangers, named Bonnie (a friend of my sister) and Dorothy (of the St. Mark of the Evangelist's shawl ministry and a friend of my mom), who graciously gifted me two of the most beautiful shawls which offered me comfort during my recovery and motivation while writing this book, I thank you. I felt your love in every loop. Your compassion is commendable and touched my heart.

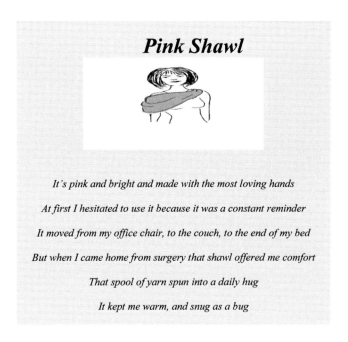

It's pink and bright and made with the most loving hands

At first I hesitated to use it because it was a constant reminder

It moved from my office chair, to the couch, to the end of my bed

But when I came home from surgery that shawl offered me comfort

That spool of yarn spun into a daily hug

It kept me warm, and snug as a bug

To my children (Ali and Jack), I am thankful for your unconditional love. Where life once stood still, I can now look forward with enthusiasm; instead of back with fear…I am thrilled at the prospect of celebrating life's greatest joys with you in the future. I am privileged every day to be your mom and fortunate you don't let me sweat the small stuff! 😊

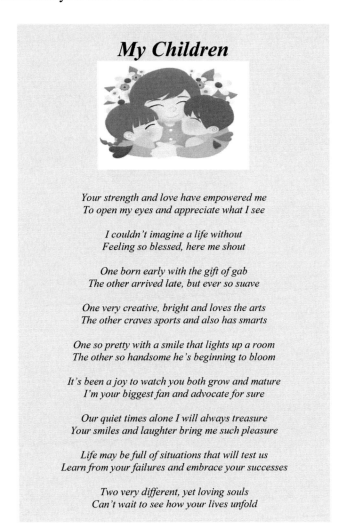

My Children

*Your strength and love have empowered me
To open my eyes and appreciate what I see*

*I couldn't imagine a life without
Feeling so blessed, here me shout*

*One born early with the gift of gab
The other arrived late, but ever so suave*

*One very creative, bright and loves the arts
The other craves sports and also has smarts*

*One so pretty with a smile that lights up a room
The other so handsome he's beginning to bloom*

*It's been a joy to watch you both grow and mature
I'm your biggest fan and advocate for sure*

*Our quiet times alone I will always treasure
Your smiles and laughter bring me such pleasure*

*Life may be full of situations that will test us
Learn from your failures and embrace your successes*

*Two very different, yet loving souls
Can't wait to see how your lives unfold*

And lastly, to my husband (Dean) …life has tested us in so many ways over the last year, I am eternally grateful for your endless love. You were and are an amazing partner, and I'm fortunate to have you on my team. You're a thoughtful, passionate and wise man. Thank you for teaching me to slow down and take notice of a world that I've spent so long rushing past.

My Love

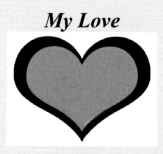

From the first time we met, I could tell
You had me at "hello"...I was under your spell

Your beauty is so much more than skin deep
An attribute I will cherish and keep

From around the world, to right back home
There's no one else I'd rather roam

Our love knows no boundaries, much like the ocean
It works do to commitment, respect and mutual devotion

You're my best guy, and my closest friend
You're the one I love to share good news with and will come to for advice
till the very end

When life wears me out, and I am really down
I find shelter in your arms, the storms seem to dissipate and expunge my frown

You know me better than anyone, and love me anyway
You're the handsome man that thrills me, whose smile brightens my days

Through good times and bad, you've always been great
To protect, honor, and love... words that will continue to define our fate

It has been nothing but extraordinary to be your wife
You're my soul mate for life

I have loved you from the very start
And will continue...till death do us part

Helpful Tips

Helpful Tips

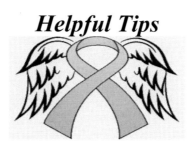

    Be your own advocate! No one will fight for you more than yourself. No question is a "dumb" question when it comes to your own body, overall health, and insurance coverage.

    Check your breasts! Be diligent doing both self-exams and annual mammograms, especially if you've already had a scare and/or breast cancer runs in your family.

    Are you dense? This is not meant to be an insult, but rather it's an organization working to push Congress to advance laws to help women understand the type of breast density they have in order to help with better mammogram testing for earlier detection of breast cancer. If you're not aware of this organization and what it means for your health, check it out…www.areyoudense.org.

Helpful Tips

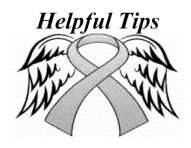

Know your breast density! In 2014, some states implemented a law requiring mammography reports sent to patients and their physicians provide an assessment of your breast density. There are 4 categories: A. Predominantly fatty; B. Scattered fibrograndular; C. Heterogeneously dense; and D. Extremely dense. The same law may require insurance carriers to pay for supplemental (i.e. MRI, 3-D mammogram, ultrasound) testing. Approximately 10% of all women have extremely dense breasts. Ask your physician what category you fall into and if your state offers the same assessment. (As of this publication, 24 states have implemented this law.)

Helpful Tips

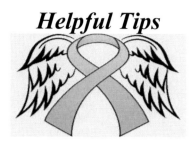

More on breast density: Some potential questions to ask your physician...

- Do I have dense breasts?
- What affects the density of my breasts?
- What screening test(s) should I get?
- How often should I have this test(s)?
- If my family members have dense breasts, will I have dense breasts too?
- What can I do to lower my risk of getting breast cancer?
- Should I be tested for the BRCA1 and BRCA2 gene mutations?

*Be sure to inquire with your insurance company prior to scheduling any tests to determine what may/ may not be covered.

Helpful Tips

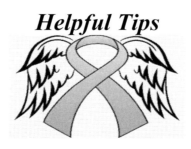

According to the American Cancer Society, signs of breast cancer are: 1. Swelling of all or part of the breast; 2. Skin irritation or dimpling; 3. Breast pain; 4. Nipple pain or turning inward; 5. Redness, scaliness, or thickening of the nipple or breast skin; 6. Nipple discharge other than breast milk; 7. A lump in the underarm area. These can be signs of less serious conditions too (i.e. infection, cyst), but it's important to get checked promptly by a doctor.

If your 3-D mammogram, ultrasound, and/or MRI suggest that there is an area(s) that requires a biopsy for further analysis, don't be alarmed if they mention inserting a clip after they extract a tissue sample. It's for your benefit, so they can keep a closer watch on that area during future tests (i.e. mammograms). And while they may quote you a 3-5 day turnaround, request that the doctor mark your sample STAT, so the lab delivers your results quicker.

Helpful Tips

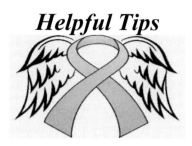

🪶 After a biopsy, the doctor or nurse should advise you on how to treat the area. For example, they may suggest ice packs for 20 minutes on/off for the first 24 hours along with some ibuprofen. Heed their advice as it will help with swelling and bruising.

🪶 Be patient with yourself. Physically, mentally, and emotionally you need time to absorb what's happening. Don't make decisions without having fully processed everything. That includes educating yourself, surrounding yourself with a support system, and being able to ask for help from objective people who care for you.

🪶 Have a companion accompany you to all of your appointments and bring a journal. Fill that journal with questions and answers about your diagnosis, treatment options, appointment dates, etc.

Helpful Tips

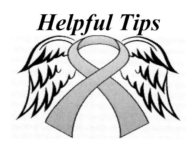

Should you get a 2nd opinion? Don't be afraid of alienating your doctor. It's okay to get a 2nd opinion. Be upfront with your initial doctor. Any professional will not see it as being disloyal, but will understand that it's your body, and ultimately **you** will make the final decisions for your treatment.

Upon diagnosis it would be helpful to check with your insurance company to see if a case worker will be assigned to you throughout your treatment. If so, it will make things much easier for you to be able to contact the same person when you need to inquire about what procedures (i.e. biopsies, MRIs, genetic tests, hospital stay & surgery, Onco tests), post-surgery visits/ therapies (i.e. home nursing care, occupational therapy, physical therapy), etc. will be covered. If not, be sure to check on every test, etc. prior to the date of service to be sure it will be covered and at what percentage. The last thing a patient needs is added stress.

Helpful Tips

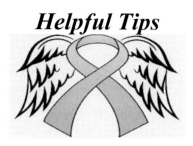

Care vs. Convenience: you may need to weigh your options and priorities. Can you afford to travel further for potentially better or more "reputable" care? Or, perhaps you need to stay closer to home because of family and/or work commitments and getting good care will work out just as well. Also, insurance will need to be a factor as to what providers are available to you, as well as, your costs for coverage. This is your health at risk and it will be a lengthy process, so be diligent in researching your doctors, hospitals, benefits, etc.

Build a network: Make a connection with a friend, family member, or colleague that has endured a similar battle. Although each individual's situation is different, you'll be able to lean on that person for questions, guidance and support when you need to talk to someone who can relate to your situation. Additionally, you might want to consider joining a support group or pursue individual counseling.

Helpful Tips

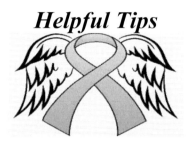

Create a keepsake box for cards, a special folder for emails and text messages...on your most difficult days these words of inspiration from family & friends will pick you up and carry you through another day.

"What's for dinner tonight?" Make and freeze a few dinners in advance of your operation. It will make your hospital stay a little less stressful from having to worry about family at home.

During recuperation, let a local friend or family member take the lead in coordinating meals (i.e. delivery, a dine out, or provide a gift card to a favorite family restaurant).

Helpful Tips

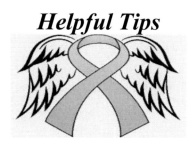

    Eat Well! Cancer patients may not need to radically change their eating habits. There is a book called Eating Well through Cancer - Easy recipes & recommendations during and after treatment (by Holly Clegg & Gerald Miletello, M.D.). Simply "Google" it and you'll find several distributors of the book. The recipes are easy & yummy! They're broken down into sections depending upon where you are with treatment and/or side-effects. Bon Appétit!

    Stages of cancer…Based on four main characteristics: the size of the cancer, whether it's invasive or non-invasive, whether it is in the lymph nodes, and whether it has spread to other parts of the body beyond the breasts. The stage of one's cancer is usually expressed on a scale from 0 to IV. The stage of cancer will help your doctor understand your prognosis and determine the best course of treatment.

Helpful Tips

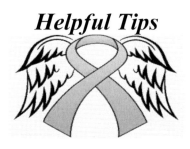

Breast reconstruction…Depending on your lifestyle and what solution might work best to fit your needs, there are surgical options as well as non-surgical options. The non-surgical options would consist of either an external breast form designed to fit inside a bra or a custom prosthesis made to stick to the skin. As for surgical procedures, they range from inserting an implant to utilizing tissue and muscle from other parts of your body (i.e. stomach, back, thigh, buttock area). It's important to understand the pros and cons of each and which option might be best for your body type.

Before making any final decisions ask your reconstruction doctor to show you "before" vs. "after" pictures so you know what to expect. You will have to live with the final result so it's important that you're comfortable with the procedure as well as your doctor's experience.

Helpful Tips

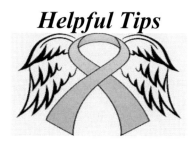

Post-surgery you may have a drains that will need to be tended to. To secure them in place you might want to use a mastectomy bra or camisole. They can be purchased at some of the larger retail stores (i.e. Nordstrom's), some local lingerie boutiques, and on-line (i.e. TLCdirect.com). Another (very inexpensive) option is a canvas construction belt (that is usually used to hold tools). They can be found at any hardware store for about $1. Wearing button down shirts will make accessing the drains much easier too.

More on drains… Be diligent in emptying them and keeping a log of when and how much fluid was emptied. This will assist your medical team with deciding when to remove your drains. In addition, if you have drains removed after surgery, you might want to wear a shirt that offers compression or a rib belt to keep from retaining fluid. While it's common to have to drain such fluid, it can be uncomfortable.

Helpful Tips

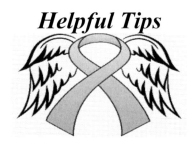

Some helpful tools post-surgery…

A. Bottom buddy wiper- Do to upper body swelling it may be difficult to reach and clean your bottom the same way you did pre-surgery when going to the bathroom. This issue will more than likely be temporary, but know that there is a solution.

B. Electric razor- Raising your arms to shave with a manual razor could be a challenge for a bit of time. Try sitting and simply raising your arm just enough to use an electric razor. It may just do the trick!

C. Folding lotion applicator- If you have hard to reach scars from surgery, it may be helpful to use a folding applicator tool to apply scar crème.

D. Button down shirts- Do to under arm swelling and a limited range of arm motion, it will be much easier to wear button down shirts for the first few weeks.

E. Step stool- To help you reach easier into cabinets.

Helpful Tips

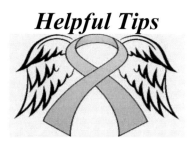

🪶 Post-surgery medication(s) might make you constipated. Try sticking to a high fiber diet and/ or taking a laxative to provide some relief.

🪶 Consider a chemo buddy…It might be helpful to have a chemo buddy (even two or three) to help accompany you to your treatments. Having a spouse, friend or family member rotate days with you will help pass the time.

🪶 If you should require chemo, ask a friend, family member, or your hairstylist to help you select a wig… someone who will give you their honest opinion. There are companies on-line, but you may want to check out local wig shops and/or vendor/flea markets in your area to try them on for size. Sometimes it's not about the price, but what makes you look and feel your best!!

Helpful Tips

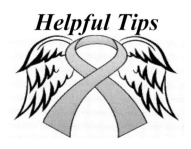

More on wigs…check out The Wig Exchange in the Westchester County area in New York. Wigs can be quite costly, especially if they're real hair vs. synthetic and quite often insurance doesn't cover the expense. If you wish to donate or borrow a wig, you can find the company on-line at www.thewigexchange.org.

Patients who endure chemotherapy treatment sometimes lose their eyebrows and eyelashes in addition to their hair. Treat yourself to a makeover at either a makeup counter in a large retail store or a smaller cosmetic boutique and learn how to pencil in your eyebrows or even wear false eyelashes. This could be a fun girls' day out too!

Helpful Tips

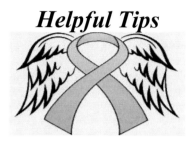

Promoting hair growth after chemotherapy...

A. A widely used remedy is olive oil. Take a capful or two and massage the oil directly into the scalp and let it sit for 30 minutes to an hour. Warm coconut oil or caster oil may be used as well. Natural aloe juice extracted from the plant or from a pure organic gel may also be used directly on the scalp.

B. Eating a balanced diet is essential.

C. You might want to supplement your diet with a vitamin B complex formula. Amino acids are also an essential aspect of growing healthy hair, so look for these and other botanicals in shampoo.

D. Ask your hairstylist to recommend products that may promote re-growth & restore luster to your hair.

E. Use warm to cool water as hot water may damage hair follicles.

*Be patient as it could be a few weeks to a few months.

Helpful Tips

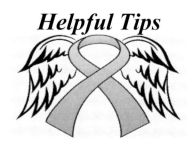

How to handle your thermostat…yes, hot flashes! Menopause can be brought on early and quickly by cancer treatments (i.e. chemo, hormone therapy). One minute your freezing and the next dripping wet. What can you do? First, try to pinpoint your hot flash triggers and patterns. Keep a record as to when they occur, what you're doing at the time, and what makes them subside. Tell your doctor too.

Avoid potential triggers, such as: smoking, caffeine, alcohol, spicy foods, weight gain, heavy materials or bulky clothes, avoid "hot" situations (i.e. hot showers),and try to reduce your stress level.

Cool off by: dressing in thin layers, keeping ice water on hand to stay well hydrated, lowering room temperature, trying a cool shower, using relaxation techniques (i.e. yoga, meditation), and diet changes.

Helpful Tips

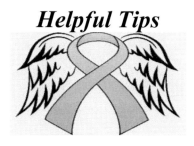

"Mind fog" (aka. Chemo brain)...what is it? Many people treated for cancer notice significant problems with their ability to manage daily mental thoughts (i.e. memory, the expression of thoughts & feelings, and processing information). The condition is poorly understood; therefore, it lacks a formal medical name and definition, and it can occur with no connection to chemotherapy. Generally, the more treatments you have, the likelihood it will put you at a higher risk. Early research indicators show that it can be brought on by chemotherapy, hormonal changes, radiation, as well as emotional stress. The good news is that most cases of "mind fog" disappear over time, anywhere from 6-12 months.

Helpful Tips

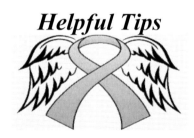

 "Mind fog"...how to deal with it?

A. Seek medical advice (possible medications)
B. Know your limitations (slow down and rest)
C. Seek help through various organizations (i.e. Breastcancer.org)
D. Use memory aids (Note cards or calendar)
E. Build brainpower (exercise your body as well as your mind by reading and singing)

Feeling like you're walking on pins & needles or getting stung by bees? It can be a common issue with nerves in your arms & legs due to chemotherapy treatment called Neuropathy. Once the treatment has stopped, this can be a lingering side effect for a few months to possibly a year. If the pain becomes intolerable, talk to your doctor.

Helpful Tips

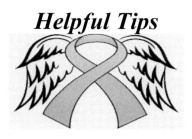

Project Chemo Crochet is a non-profit organization that sends support to those battling cancer in the form of a crocheted blanket. Each blanket is made with love to comfort those in the fight. If you would like to participate in this cause, order a blanket for someone, or make a donation to this worthy cause, please go to the link: http://projectchemocrochet.com.

Clean for a Reason...a non-profit organization that offers free house cleaning services for cancer patients. This could be a great gift idea or a patient can fill out an application themselves. Their website identifies participating maid services by State and accepts donations.

Helpful Tips

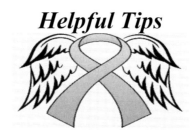

One's journey with breast cancer does not end after their initial surgery. Quite often there is some form of follow up treatment (i.e. chemo, radiation, medication, another surgery). It can be a lengthy, painful and daunting process. If you have a friend or family member going through it, reach out to them every few weeks to let them know you're thinking of them and wishing them well. A simple text, email, phone call or note to let them know you care will give them strength and a helpful pick me up when they least expect it and probably need it.

From the start of one's diagnosis a notebook is a useful tool to track bills and/or receipts. When following up with a billing department, be sure to document the date, time and person you spoke with. Also, don't be afraid to question or appeal a decision by your insurance company. They make mistakes too!

Helpful Tips

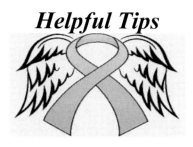

🪶 Don't forget to hug your partner. Whether it's a spouse, friend or family member that has stayed by your side throughout your journey, let them know you appreciate their support. It can be a long stressful and exhausting process for both the patient as well as those closest to you.

🪶 Find your rainbow in each day. It could be the tweet of a bird, a beautiful sunrise or sunset, rekindling an old friendship, helping someone else in need, a hug, lunch with a friend, dancing like no one is watching, holding hands with a loved one on a walk, or blasting your favorite song on the radio. As they say, take time to smell the roses…

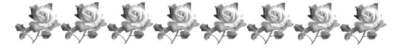

Available Resources

The following list provides a small sample of links to organizations that offer the latest information about breast cancer research, statistics, services and products for breast cancer patients.

Breast Cancer Causes, Symptoms & Treatments:
American Cancer Society (www.cancer.org/cancer/breastcancer)

Breastcancer.org (www.breastcancer.org)

Dr. Susan Love Research Foundation (www.drsusanloveresearch.org)

National Institute of Cancer (www.cancer.gov/types/breast)

*Note: Several large research hospitals have their own websites which provide additional information about trials and research in progress.

Community Support:
Are you dense? (www.areyoudense.org)

Gilda's Club (websites vary by location)

Living Beyond Breast Cancer (www.lbbc.org)

Susan G. Komen (ww5.komen.org)

Services/ Products:
American Cancer Society's Tender Loving Care – Offers cancer products – wigs, bras, etc. (www.TLCdirect.com)

Clean for a Reason – Offers free house cleaning services for patients (www.cleanforareason.org)

Greater Good Stores – Sell pink ribbon items that fund screening and research (http://thebreastcancersite.greatergood.com)

Pink Ribbon Store – Sell pink ribbon items which help fund screening (www.pinkribbonstore.com)

Project Chemo Crochet – Donate crocheted blankets to patients (http://projectchemocrochet.com)

The Wig Exchange – Accepts and loans wigs (www.thewigexchange.org)

Journal

If you were recently diagnosed with breast cancer, perhaps you will find keeping notes in your own journal helpful during your treatment. The following pages have been designed to capture doctors' appointments and important discussion points. In the beginning, there will be so much information being discussed that you will want to have notes to reference as it comes time to make crucial decisions about your treatment.

Date: **Time:**

Doctor:

Patient's Questions:

Key Remarks:

Next Appointment -
Date: **Time:**

Date: **Time:**

Doctor:

Patient's Questions:

Key Remarks:

Next Appointment -
Date: **Time:**

Date: **Time:**

Doctor:

Patient's Questions:

Key Remarks:

Next Appointment -
Date: **Time:**

Date: **Time:**

Doctor:

Patient's Questions:

Key Remarks:

Next Appointment -
Date: **Time:**

Date: **Time:**

Doctor:

Patient's Questions:

Key Remarks:

Next Appointment -
Date: **Time:**

Pink Warrior Poetry & Tips

Date: **Time:**

Doctor:

Patient's Questions:

Key Remarks:

Next Appointment -
Date: **Time:**

Date: **Time:**

Doctor:

Patient's Questions:

Key Remarks:

Next Appointment -
Date: **Time:**

Date: **Time:**

Doctor:

Patient's Questions:

Key Remarks:

Next Appointment -
Date: **Time:**

Date: **Time:**

Doctor:

Patient's Questions:

Key Remarks:

Next Appointment -
Date: **Time:**

Date: **Time:**

Doctor:

Patient's Questions:

Key Remarks:

Next Appointment -
Date: **Time:**

Date: **Time:**

Doctor:

Patient's Questions:

Key Remarks:

Next Appointment -
Date: **Time:**

Date: **Time:**

Doctor:

Patient's Questions:

Key Remarks:

Next Appointment -
Date: **Time:**

Date: **Time:**

Doctor:

Patient's Questions:

Key Remarks:

Next Appointment -
Date: **Time:**

Pink Warrior Poetry & Tips

Date: **Time:**

Doctor:

Patient's Questions:

Key Remarks:

Next Appointment -
Date: **Time:**

Date: **Time:**

Doctor:

Patient's Questions:

Key Remarks:

Next Appointment -
Date: **Time:**

Date: **Time:**

Doctor:

Patient's Questions:

Key Remarks:

Next Appointment -
Date: **Time:**

Date: **Time:**

Doctor:

Patient's Questions:

Key Remarks:

Next Appointment -
Date: **Time:**

Date: **Time:**

Doctor:

Patient's Questions:

Key Remarks:

Next Appointment -
Date: **Time:**

Date: **Time:**

Doctor:

Patient's Questions:

Key Remarks:

Next Appointment -
Date: **Time:**

May there be hope for the fighters, peace for the survivors and prayers for the taken.

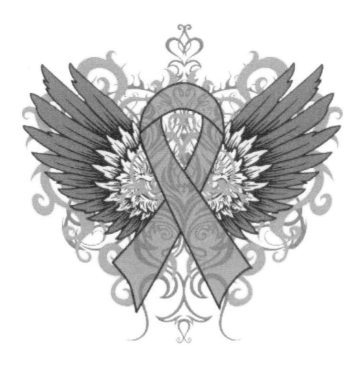

Made in United States
North Haven, CT
27 October 2021